What's Right For Me?

Making decisions in pregnancy and childbirth

Second edition

Dr Sara Wickham

What's Right For Me?
Making decisions in pregnancy and childbirth
Second edition published 2018 by Birthmoon Creations
© 2018 Sara Wickham
www.sarawickham.com

ISBN-10: 1999806417
ISBN-13: 978-1999806415
Also available as an e-book

This book offers general information for interest only and does not
constitute or replace individualised professional midwifery or medical care
and advice. Whilst every effort has been made to ensure the accuracy and
currency of the information herein, the author accepts no liability or
responsibility for any loss or damage caused, or thought to be caused, by
making decisions based upon the information in this book and recommends
that you use it in conjunction with other trusted sources of information.

Acknowledgements

I have the best friends and colleagues, whose support and expertise helps make my books and other work possible. A big thank you to all of those who helped facilitate the birth of this book, especially Beverley Beech, Gill Boden, Nadine Edwards, Julie Frohlich, Chris Hackforth, Kirsten Small, Hannah Souter and Debbie Willett.

I also want to acknowledge the work of Dr Kate Granger and her husband Chris Pointon, founders of the #hellomynameis campaign. During her experience of having cancer, Kate noticed that many hospital staff did not introduce themselves before giving care. She began the #hellomynameis campaign on social media as a means of reminding healthcare staff of the importance of introductions as a cornerstone of person-centred and compassionate health care. Kate's husband Chris has kept the campaign alive since Kate's death in 2016. The #hellomynameis campaign has always resonated with my own passion in this area. I have borrowed Kate's phrase for a chapter heading in this book and want to encourage any health care professional who isn't already aware of this campaign to seek more information at https://hellomynameis.org.uk/

About the Author

Dr Sara Wickham PhD, RM, MA, PGCert, BA(Hons) is a midwife, educator, writer and researcher who works independently, dividing her working time between speaking, writing, teaching online courses and live workshops, consulting and creating resources for midwives and birth workers.

Sara's career has been varied; she has lived and worked in the UK, the USA and New Zealand, edited three professional journals and lectured in more than twenty-five countries.

You can find Sara online at www.sarawickham.com, where she writes a twice weekly blog and a free monthly newsletter. Some of her work is also shared at www.facebook.com/saramidwife and @DrSaraWickham

Also by Sara Wickham

Anti-D in Midwifery: panacea or paradox?
Appraising Research into Childbirth
Birthing Your Placenta (with Nadine Edwards)
Group B Strep Explained
Inducing Labour: making informed decisions
Midwifery Best Practice (volumes 1-5)
Sacred Cycles: the spiral of women's wellbeing
Vitamin K and the Newborn
101 Tips for planning, writing and surviving your dissertation

Contents

1. Introduction

The decisions that we make shape our experiences, health and lives.

The decisions that we make about pregnancy and childbirth can have particularly long lasting effects on our experiences, health and lives, as well as on those of our children and families. But many of the decisions which women need to make on their childbearing journey are complex, confusing and sometimes overwhelming. They are often made harder by the fact that we live in a world which is filled with information, options and opinions; not all of which are very woman-centred.

This book has been written to try to help people make more sense of pregnancy and birth-related decisions, and it is my hope that it might help you to make the ones that are right for you. I'll talk you through some ways of thinking about information and give you some background knowledge which I hope might be helpful as you navigate the decision-making landscape. But, because one of the things that I am going to suggest to you in here is to find out about the source of the information before you decide whether it is of value to you, please allow me to begin by introducing myself and telling you where I am coming from.

Hello, my name is Sara

I'm a midwife who has cared for many women and families and attended the births of hundreds of babies in birth centres, hospitals and their own homes. My passion is in helping women and their families to get the information and support they need so they can make the decisions that are right for them. I've written several books with this aim, and I run a website and blog offering information to anyone who would like to stop by. I'm also an educator and a researcher. I teach health care professionals and birth workers; helping

1

them stay up-to-date with the evidence.

I don't have a hidden agenda in my work. I have a very clear one, and I'd like to spell out where I stand and why I have written this book.

Firstly, I know that women and babies are great at giving birth and being born. I know that women's bodies are immensely capable of growing a baby and giving birth physiologically, and I know from experience that the majority of women will give birth without problems and with happy and healthy outcomes if we create the right circumstances for their labour and birth. That's what I have focused on for most of my career as a practising midwife.

But I also know that the birth journey can be unpredictable and things don't always go to plan. I have supported many women and families as they have needed to move from their 'plan A' (that is, what happens if everything goes well and they go into labour and progress without any major issues), to plan B (which is about what they would want and what would be important to them if an issue occurs and a change in plan is needed) or even plan C (or what they would want in the event of a major issue or change of plan, such as where a woman ended up needing a caesarean section). A small number of women will need help for themselves or their baby no matter how much we plan or set the scene to be optimal, and then there are women like my friend Colleen, who plan to have their baby in the hospital, only to find that they have a fast labour and end up birthing their baby at home. What makes the difference in these situations is that women and families have had the chance to explore these possibilities beforehand and think through what is important for them. The sense of inner power that women gain from taking responsibility for their own birthing journey and for the decisions that they make on that journey is immense, even if things don't go quite as anticipated.

Not everyone will want the same thing, of course. People want all sorts of different things, and I wholeheartedly celebrate that difference. But even more than that, I champion every woman's right to think about and decide what is right for her. Women are more than capable of making the decisions that are right for them and their babies, and healthcare workers need to understand that!

But many women do not realise that all pregnancy and birth decisions are theirs to make. Some are not prepared for the nature or scale of the decisions that they will face. And I have seen too many women and families struggle because they haven't had the time, opportunity or space to think about what they would want, or to think about how the decisions that they are making may be shaped and affected by some of the aspects of our rapidly changing culture.

This is how I see the problem

A number of features of our modern culture have made making birth-related decisions trickier than ever. Our TV, cinema and computer screens are filled with dramatic and unrealistic portrayals of birth, which often make it out to be 'risky' and cause people to feel scared of it. Such programmes also give people unrealistic ideas about labour and birth. A good example here is how, in TV and films, labour is often shown as being much shorter than it is in real life. This can then make it difficult for women who do not realise that they may spend a good many hours in what midwives call 'early labour' before their labour is considered to be 'established' or progressing. Some of these women will end up with intervention that they did not want, which they probably didn't need and which might have been prevented if they had been able to gain a more realistic sense of what labour and birth can be like.

Social media feeds can easily become full of negative images, judgements and people telling others what to think and do. We live in a consumer culture and there exist people and companies who have an interest in perpetuating fear and persuading people to make the choices that are right for the company, because it benefits them personally or financially.

And we have created centralised and standardised health care systems, which tend to offer a 'one size fits all' approach. In such systems, people can feel they are on a conveyor belt and professionals feel overworked and unable to give individualised care. Such systems leave many people feeling disrespected, dissatisfied and hurt, not to mention physically and/or emotionally traumatised.

A related issue is that nowadays many women don't have confidence in their own bodies. For too long, women have been told that their bodies are the wrong shape and size, that they're too hairy, too dirty, too smelly, too old, too fat and that they don't work properly. We hear and see constant (though often very subtle) messages telling us that we are 'inadequate' and deficient and that we grow the wrong sized babies. We have been convinced that our bodies aren't trustworthy enough to be allowed to labour without being closely monitored and watched; even though being monitored and watched can slow down our labours. We hear that we don't go into labour at the right time, that we don't labour quickly enough or well enough and then, when our babies do come out, we're told that we then don't have enough milk to feed them. Somewhat paradoxically, and despite all these criticisms, we also receive the message that a woman's body is for the enjoyment of others rather than herself. Is it any wonder that many women don't know how to trust their bodies or have a sense that decisions about their body are theirs and theirs alone to make?

In the months and years after they give birth, many women say that they wished that they had explored different options or had had more information about other paths that might have been available to them. Some women, for instance, wish they had chosen a different kind of caregiver or a different place of birth. Or that they had not agreed to something that was offered. Or that they had asked for something else.

Others are really happy with the choices that they made. The reality is that, for healthy women who live in high income countries today, many birth decisions are equally safe and appropriate. We know, for instance, that most women and babies are just as safe no matter whether birth takes place at home, in a birth centre or in hospital (Birthplace in England Collaborative Group 2011). We are also learning that, even when research tells us that one option may be slightly safer than another on a population basis (that is, when we consider what works for large numbers of women and babies across the board), that doesn't necessarily make it better for an individual woman or baby. We also often see that, even when there appears to be a relative difference between two possible courses of action (or inaction), the absolute difference between these options turns out to be quite small.

But these nuances and complexities often get lost when we reduce everything to likes, comments and retweets and when rushed conversations take place in what can feel like a noisy, crowded marketplace. It's clear that we need to find a way to get away from the noise so that we can talk about these issues, and to help people think about things before they make some of the most important decisions of their lives.

Getting away from the noise

When I was on holiday with my husband Chris a few years ago, he and I walked through a Greek marketplace near a major tourist destination very early one morning. When we set out, the market was waking up, but it didn't take long to turn into a symphony of sound and activity. The local merchants unpacked and spread their wares, erected sunshades, began to brew gorgeous-smelling coffee and exchanged news with their neighbours. The locals started arriving to buy the coffee, followed by more tourists like us. Within a short space of time, the symphony had reached a crescendo, and we found ourselves feeling overwhelmed and unable to think straight!

Chris spotted a gateway into the cool walled gardens of a museum, and we went through it. It was a beautiful hidden sanctuary of peace and cooling breezes. We sat on a bench amongst the ancient walls and the fragrant, sun-soaked herbs and it was as if we had entered a different world.

I sometimes think that the birth decision arena has become a bit like that marketplace. We are faced with this constant onslaught of images, ideas, opinions and judgements about what we should and shouldn't be doing. And my hope is that this book might serve as the equivalent of the bench in that cool, walled garden. You might rest, read and decide that you really want to go back through the marketplace and buy everything! Or you might decide to look for another way out of the museum garden, or take a different path or do something else that you've never previously considered. In this book, I am merely offering you the chance to rest awhile and ponder.

I'm also offering some background knowledge about what's out there, and about the different perspectives that people take in relation to birth. Because one of the things that makes birth-related decisions tricky is that there *are* different perspectives out there. Another complicating factor is the way that the concept of risk is used to try to get people to 'buy' one idea over another. In this book, I'll talk you through all those things and more. I'll share and discuss some tools which can help you think through what is already important to you and your family, and I'll walk you through some of the key elements of the different decisions you might need to make.

I'm not going to outline the pros and cons of every decision that you might encounter. Even if I wanted to or had room for that, the issues differ in relation to personal factors, where you live, who is around you, your health and beliefs, your previous experiences and who you are as a person. There is also lots of information out there on particular situations from different perspectives and, once you've read this book, I hope you'll be better equipped to look for the different perspectives and deeper information in relation to any decision.

At its heart, then, this book is about helping people to be

in a better place to make their own decisions. No matter whether you want the modern norm or something alternative, whether you want to aim for an undisturbed birth or while attached to all available technology, this book aims to offer lots of food for thought so that you can consider and decide what's right for you. The first few chapters offer some general information designed to help you get a sense of what the landscape (for want of a better metaphor) of birth decision making actually looks like. That is, I'm going to explain some of the different perspectives that people take towards birth and some of the bigger issues which influence our culture so you can better understand the 'lie of the land'. The chapters in the second half of the book offer some theoretical and practical tips; tools and ways of thinking that I hope will help you to navigate that landscape in order to find the path that's right for you. Then there's a resources section which offers ideas for further reading and a series of appendices with specific information and suggestions about a few key areas.

So please make yourself comfortable, put your feet up, and let's pour you a cup of tea...

Sara Wickham. Wiltshire, England. Spring 2018.

2. What does the childbirth decision making landscape look like?

Many women don't realise how many decisions they need to make during their pregnancy, birth and parenting years. This is understandable, because some of these decisions aren't widely discussed in society. Many people live in smaller and less tightly-knit families than in the past, so we are less likely to experience our mothers and other relatives being pregnant with other children. We also face many more decisions today than we did even twenty years ago because the options and available technology have increased. And some of the most important decisions may not even be offered as decisions.

Psychologists have helped us understand that, often, the decisions we make are not based on a rational weighing up of the options. Sometimes, we simply follow what we see others doing. That works really well for some people and in some situations, but not for others. I often advise women and families to try to identify and then put aside the assumptions that they grew up with and consider what they would really like or want. Just because it's the fashion right now (or it's what your sister did) doesn't mean it's the right decision for you and your family. On the other hand, just because no-one else in your friendship group has done something, doesn't mean you shouldn't be the first.

Here are some examples of the key decisions that you might need to make during the childbearing year.

Where would you like to have your baby? Home, birth centre, hospital or somewhere else?

Many women in high income countries now grow up assuming that they will give birth in hospital, and perhaps believing that hospital is the safest place to give birth. That's perhaps inevitable, as this is what we see most commonly on TV, on the internet and in other forms of media. But there are other options and, as I mentioned above, research shows that, for healthy women, giving birth at home or in a birth centre are equally safe (Birthplace in England Collaborative Group 2011). Lower-tech environments are known to be associated with fewer interventions and women who give birth at home or in homelike settings with midwives tend to have more positive feelings about their birth experiences. But there are pros and cons to all settings, so it's important to think about what's right for you and your family.

Who would you like to have with you during your labour and birth? (Midwife, partner, family, children, obstetrician, doula, friend, others?)

It can also be important to think about what support you want during your labour and birth and who can best give you that. These days, we tend to assume that our partners will be with us during birth, but that hasn't always been the case and it isn't right for all couples. Some women like to have their mum or a friend present, while others think that's a terrible idea. The same goes for having older children present. This is often easier to arrange in an out-of-hospital setting, but you can ask if this is possible if you are planning a hospital birth and this is important to you. It can be a good way of finding out how flexible a place is going to be in meeting your needs.

Another important and related question is which birth professional(s) will best be able to support you and help you get what you want. And by 'what you want', I mean what you consider to be the safest, most appropriate kind of care and situation that will meet your needs and enable you to birth safely, bond with your baby and experience a journey that feels right and good for you and your family. Because this experience, as I said right at the beginning, has the potential to affect you for a very long time.

What kind of birth experience would you prefer – and what can you do to maximise your chances of having that experience?

I'm not going to suggest for a moment that you can truly plan out your birth experience or that it will be exactly as you imagine, because that would be unhelpful and unrealistic. I've already said that the birth journey can be unpredictable, and very few women have the exact experience they think they will. But that shouldn't stop you from thinking about what's important to you and putting in place whatever you can to support your preferences and maximise the chance of things going as you hope. Again, it can be useful to have a plan A (for if everything goes as you hope), a plan B (what is most important to you if a plan change is needed) and a plan C (what you would want in the event of a major plan change).

When people are able to think about what they would want in those different scenarios and what is important to them, then the factors that I've already mentioned, such as the setting and the people that you choose for your birth, may fall into place easily. If you know you want an epidural, you'll need a hospital which offers that service. If you want to have your baby in hospital but the most important thing to you is that your partner never has to leave your side, you'll want to ask around and look at whether and how this is possible locally, both in the scenario of plan A (you go into hospital in labour and go straight to the labour ward, where partners are generally welcome) and plan B (you decide to have your labour induced, in which case you may find the situation is very different with regards to your partner staying with you).

Sometimes you'll need to take an extra step to put what you need in place. If your plan A is a home birth with your children around you and a family-sized birth pool, then you'll want a skilled, confident midwife who is comfortable with those things and who clearly believes in your ability to give birth in your own power. Plus, of course, a means of getting the pool, which might be a via a friend or family member, through your midwife or doula, from a birth-related centre or charity or maybe as the result of an appeal to friends of friends on social media.

If you are allocated to or have engaged a midwife or doctor who doesn't seem confident in your ability to birth, then trust your instincts and reconsider your options. Depending on where you are in the world and how care is structured, you might need to change care provider, ask for another midwife or doctor, consider hiring a private midwife, or engage a friend or doula to support you as well. Appendices 1 and 2 offer ideas and resources to help with this.

Do you want to have routine screening tests and interventions during your pregnancy and labour? Are there any you particularly want to have or to avoid?

Another feature of modern, high-income countries is that health services tend to make recommendations about what should and should not be offered to all pregnant or birthing women. These recommendations then influence what you are told will happen when you enter the maternity services. But all pregnant and birthing women are not the same, and you may prefer to make decisions based upon your unique and personal situation. Or, of course, you might decide you want to follow population-level recommendations – that's a perfectly reasonable decision as well. Later, I'll guide you through the types of interventions you may be offered so that you'll know what that part of the landscape looks like too.

Do you want to do things to optimise your well-being and that of your baby, even if it means looking for information and opportunities over and above that which you'll get in the maternity care system?

Because systems of maternity care are looking after so many women and babies, the advice they give tends to be basic and standardised. So within these care systems, the decisions that you will be offered are often more about deciding whether to stick with the norm or opt out of routine intervention. You might not always be given information on additional things that you can do which may help make a positive difference for you and your baby or babies.

A good example of this is nutrition. You may receive basic, standard nutritional advice from the maternity services, but many midwives and healers who work outside of the system (who have more time to spend with women) give highly detailed and tailored information about how women can optimise their health in general and nutrition in particular.

Other areas of wellness that are available but not necessarily offered within standard maternity care include pregnancy yoga, other types of pregnancy-focused exercise and fitness activity, bodywork, alternative therapies and a whole range of educational and social opportunities which offer different approaches to preparing for birth and parenting, such as classes focused around yoga, mindfulness or hypnosis-based approaches. Some of these are offered as a private service, but there are often ways for those on a low income to access such services. If this is something you're interested in, it can be as simple as spending some time looking or asking around to see what's available in your area. Appendix 1 includes suggestions of the kinds of groups that you might look out for in your area.

Are there things that you particularly want for yourself and/or your baby during the birth itself?

We have learned, over the past few decades, that there are some things that we can do which will give our newborn babies a significant advantage. One example of this is skin-to-skin cuddling, which has many physiological, social and behavioural advantages for mother, baby, bonding and breastfeeding (UNICEF 2018). Another option is optimal (sometimes called delayed) cord clamping, where the cord is not clamped and cut immediately at birth. This allows the baby to get her full complement of blood before the supply is cut off. Delayed cord clamping is recommended by the World Health Organization (2018) and it is known to help ensure that babies have good iron stores. In another example, women who want to breastfeed may be keen to do this as soon as possible after birth, as we know this this optimises breastfeeding success and bonding.

If you are having your baby at home or in a birth centre, then you are more likely to find that support for these things is standard. There is more variation in hospitals, especially in some countries, so if you are planning a hospital birth and one or more of these things is important to you, it would be wise to ask questions and discuss your options ahead of time.

Do you want your baby to have screening tests and interventions when s/he is born?

Again, population-level recommendations exist about the kinds of screening tests and interventions which are offered to newborn babies, because we live at a time in which governments and professional bodies feel they need to make suggestions about what the default option should be. These recommendations vary quite a bit between countries, but they often include taking blood to test for certain conditions and offering injections of vitamin K, vaccines and, in some countries, eye drops to prevent infection.

Some people are happy to follow recommendations, and others want to look into the evidence about each one. Later, I will discuss the different kinds of interventions that are offered and offer some frameworks and tools for thinking about what is right for you and your family. You'll then be able to apply those principles to your own situation.

3. What is informed decision making?

The right of women to make informed choices about their care is, in most countries, enshrined in law as well as in the principles and policies of systems of maternity care. We have the right to decide whether or not something is done to us, and this includes procedures, drugs, screening tests (and lots more) and even whether we want to engage with a particular system of care or not. We certainly have the right to decide who gets to put their fingers or medical instruments upon or inside our bodies, and we have the right to decide whether or not we want to be in a particular place. And we have the right to decide how our babies are cared for, before and after birth, although once a baby is born this situation does become more complex, because the baby is then considered a separate person with rights of its own.

There is no universally agreed definition of what constitutes an informed decision, but I would describe an informed decision as a decision that is made by a person after careful consideration of the situation, any relevant evidence or information and in relation to their unique circumstances, beliefs and experiences. Relevant evidence or information could include your own experience or that of other women, information from books, research or other media, information from your midwife or doctor and/or your intuition or bodily knowledge. The word 'informed' also tends to imply that the person is aware of the various sides of an issue or debate (and there is often more than one way to look at an issue), rather than that she is making a decision simply because it is what is expected of her, or what the midwife or doctor recommends, or most women in that situation decide.

Informed decision-making is not about being persuaded or coerced, however nicely, into making the decision someone else thinks you should make. It's not about following norms or trends. It is not about basing important choices on just one piece of information until you find out whether that information is accurate. It is not usually about making decisions very quickly without thinking carefully through the options and discussing them with the people you care about.

Sometimes, women make decisions that are not truly informed because they don't know what information is out there. Sometimes they are too tired, stressed, sore, anxious or busy to want to engage with the issues, so they decide to go with the default option, which is another reason why it's good to find a caregiver whose ideas and beliefs are compatible with yours. For instance, when Jill was asked if she wanted her baby to have vitamin K, she asked the midwife what other women usually did. Upon hearing that the vast majority of babies received this, she decided to go with the majority and let her baby have it too. In some ways we could say that Jill's decision wasn't informed, because she didn't know all the facts for herself, but in reality some women do not want to make every tiny decision and are happy to go along with the recommendation of their caregiver in certain areas.

Be wary of those who are not open to the kind of decisions you might want to make. Be wary of people who say, *"well, if it was me"* or, *"well, if you were my wife/partner"*, unless you specifically asked them that question. You are not that person, nor that person's wife or partner, and your needs, preferences and situation are different from theirs. This kind of statement can be a sign that someone is rather paternalistic in their attitudes; they think they know what is best for you, and they may try and impose that upon you.

Most birth attendants will discuss with you the fact that there are occasionally times when making decisions may be difficult. But beware of those whose response to a discussion of the choices you want to make is always, *"let's wait and see"*. That can sometimes be a helpful and reasonable thing to say, in the sense that labour and birth aren't predictable, but it can also be a sign that they do not agree with the decisions that you want to make. If that is the case, you may find them steering you in a different direction later in pregnancy or when you are actually in labour. Not listening to women is disrespectful on the part of the caregiver. Not being listened to can be really stressful and potentially traumatising, especially as some women don't feel they have the energy to insist that their wishes are fully respected.

If your caregiver will not commit to the decisions you have made, and you do not think their explanation of this is reasonable, then you might want to explore other options. It is reasonable to make a birth plan noting your preferences and decisions ahead of time, while acknowledging that you understand that circumstances may change, or that you may feel differently when you are in labour. Again, the references, resources and reading section at the back of this book will point you in the direction of further information.

It is always worth listening to what caregivers have to say, though. It might be that they have knowledge or a perspective which is worth considering and that you weren't previously aware of. Be aware that, if you end up deciding to do something different from what is recommended, you may be asked to sign something to say that you have been given information and understood the options available to you.

Some women are very grateful that their caregiver gently challenged their ideas. Laurel read an article in a magazine that suggested (inaccurately) that having a baby by caesarean section meant she would recover more quickly. She went immediately to her obstetrician and told her she wanted an elective (planned) caesarean section. Laurel was lucky, in that she had a doctor who felt it was important to talk decisions through first, and Laurel's doctor spent a while chatting to Laurel before making her another appointment to talk to an experienced midwife. This midwife also spent a long time talking to Laurel about the different options and her hopes and expectations and Laurel ultimately decided to have her baby in the local birth centre. Laurel and her partner were delighted with their decision and Laurel is still grateful to the obstetrician who didn't take her first decision at face value.

Sheila, on the other hand, was grateful for the midwife

who talked her through the same kinds of information and ultimately supported her decision that a repeat caesarean section was the right decision for her.

Unfortunately, a few people feel so strongly that their viewpoint is the correct one that they try to scare women and families into making the decisions they think are right. They are probably doing it for what they think are good reasons, but it can be shocking and upsetting if it happens to you. So I feel compelled to tell you about this, because I don't know any other way of helping protect you from the shock of this or from the impact that it can have on the decision-making of women and families who weren't prepared for such tactics.

Coercion may be subtle or overt. It may feel like coercion or bullying, or it may involve someone teasing you, laughing at you, telling you that something is 'hospital policy' or suggesting that harm will come to you or your baby if you do (or don't do) something. Coercion may also be sugar-coated, where a professional explains very kindly and sweetly that the option or course of action they are suggesting is in your or your baby's best interests, or needs to happen.

Coercion may come from friends, family members and people in our social circles as well as professionals. You might have people around you who are subtly or overtly mocking, judging or questioning your choices. Friends, colleagues and family members may mean well, but you may need to clarify your boundaries. Some women feel hassled in an indirect way, by people they don't even know well. Sue decided, towards the end of her pregnancy, to stop using a particular social media site. She realised that she was being continually exposed to posts and pictures which were undermining her own beliefs and choices, and that this wasn't helpful to her.

If you think someone is trying to coerce you, they probably are. Remember that your decisions will affect you and your baby and family far more than they affect birth professionals or your social circle. Find a way to get away from the situation to think and seek support.

4. Perspectives on childbirth

When they have a headache, an upset stomach or a strained muscle, some people feel that taking pharmaceutical drugs is the best and easiest way to cure the problem and relieve pain, while others prefer first to explore natural or holistic options and use medication as a last resort.

It's the same with childbirth. Some people tend to trust that women's bodies have been designed or created to grow and birth babies and that it's best to use simple, holistic options first and draw upon medical treatment only if it is truly needed. Others feel that technology should be utilised at every opportunity, even if that leads to more intervention than might otherwise occur.

We know that people have different personalities and subscribe to different belief systems, ideas and values about all kinds of things: religion, politics, work, health, parenting and, of course, pregnancy and birth. A friend and colleague of mine, Robbie Davis-Floyd, described three basic belief systems (or paradigms) in relation to childbirth (2001, 2004), and I think these are a helpful way to consider this area. Robbie describes these as the technocratic, humanistic and holistic paradigms. In this chapter, I'm going to describe each and also say a few wider things about belief systems, because an understanding of this helps many people make sense of the differing information and approaches they encounter.

The technocratic approach

Within what we call the technocratic paradigm, the body is essentially viewed as a machine, and the patient as an object who is alienated from the healthcare practitioner. Diagnosis and treatment occur from the outside in, so there is a focus on the professional's use of technology to see inside the body, generally without taking account of or asking about the person's own, embodied knowledge.

Examples of this include using technologies like ultrasound and electronic fetal monitoring to monitor the baby's growth, age and wellbeing, rather than seeking information from the baby's mother. The technocratic practitioner often expects to be viewed as the expert and to make the decisions, and these decisions often focus on active or even aggressive intervention with a focus on short-term results rather than long-term or wider consequences.

Other features of the technocratic approach include a separation of mind and body and the idea that authority and responsibility lie with the professional rather than the patient. Within technocratic systems of health care, the focus is on hierarchies, standardisation and profit. Proponents of this belief system can sometimes be intolerant of other modalities (such as alternative therapies or alternative healing systems) and ways of thinking. This is the belief system that currently predominates in much of the industrialised world today.

People whose views are aligned with the technocratic approach view birth as a potentially risky event which can be considered safe only in retrospect. (We'll talk more about risk in the next chapter). They feel better when women and babies are monitored as closely and continuously as possible and they are often fearful of spontaneous, natural labour and birth, although they may or may not admit this to themselves or others. People who hold such beliefs may act on their fear by encouraging women not to make choices which they perceive as risky. They may tend (whether they realise it or not) to see women's bodies as inferior to men's, and this may cause them to blame women or their bodies when things don't go to plan. This laying of blame is often inappropriate, because there are many situations where problems are caused not by the woman's body, but by the failure of the system, or the setting or the guidelines to accommodate or account for individual variation in how women labour and give birth.

It's tempting to feel that technology must give information that is better and more accurate than a mother's own observations. But midwives, doctors and sonographers (that is, the people who perform ultrasounds) know that it's not that simple at all. The best information comes from a combination of three things. These include listening to the mother, using technology appropriately and sparingly when necessary (rather than routinely, where it can lead to over diagnosis of non-existent problems) and using other kinds of knowledge, including research evidence, experience and clinical judgement in order to assess the situation and help the woman make the right decision for her.

In my view, research evidence alone is not the answer. You will find some people claiming that birth decisions must be 'evidence-based'. And I would totally agree that research evidence can be tremendously useful in telling us certain things. But, as in the example above, research evidence is only really useful when combined with other kinds of knowledge, and it can be very limited. A recent study showed that only around 9-12% of obstetric guidelines are based on top-quality evidence (Prusova *et al* 2014). And even when top-quality evidence exists, that doesn't mean that every woman or family will want to go along with what it says.

The humanistic approach

The next belief system is called the humanistic paradigm. People who hold humanistic beliefs see the body as an organism rather than a machine, and are likely to approach a patient as a person with feelings, taking account of the context of their life. There is more of a sense of connection and caring between the person and the health care provider and humanistic people are more likely to pick up when a person is stressed, and they will want to take into account the social and psychological elements of a situation, like how someone might feel about being separated from their partner or family.

A good example of this occurs where midwives who are talking to women about possible induction of labour want to ensure the woman knows not only why this is recommended, but also about the downsides and risks of the process, which includes a good chance that the women will be separated from her partner for a day or two while she is on an antenatal ward waiting for the induction drugs to take effect.

Humanistic practitioners see the mind and body as connected and they will use both 'outside in' (e.g. ultrasound) and 'inside out' (seeking the person's knowledge) types of information in making a diagnosis and recommending treatment. Care is driven by compassion and there is an awareness about and an openness towards other modalities, such as alternative therapies. There may still be plenty of emphasis on using science and technology, but this will be employed in a more compassionate way. Information, decision-making and responsibility are shared between the practitioner and the person seeking care. People who take a humanistic approach often work in health care systems and strive to reach a balance between the needs of the system and the needs of the individual.

Those who take a humanistic approach believe that women's bodies have been designed or created to grow, birth and feed their babies and they trust that the process generally works rather well. Although they realise that occasionally things do not go to plan (and are equipped to deal with situations where help is necessary), they understand that it is good to try to eradicate fear and focus on safety, feeling that fear itself can be the cause of problems. They may still do quite a lot of monitoring and they may be in a situation where they feel compelled to 'follow the guidelines', but they will try to do this in a way that is more person-centred and friendly.

The holistic approach

Finally, we have the holistic paradigm. In this approach, the body is seen as an energy system which interacts with other energy systems, and in this there are parallels both with some schools of ancient wisdom and cutting-edge scientific disciplines such as quantum mechanics. Such wisdom presents a challenge to the technocratic approach, which is rooted in ideas such as separation, and shows that there isn't necessarily a simple, linear explanation for everything and that we might benefit from taking a wider perspective.

For those with a holistic viewpoint, the focus is on healing the whole person, often from the inside out, and within the context of their life. Individualisation of care is prioritised, and authority, decision-making power and responsibility are viewed as being the remit of the person who is seeking care or healing. Science and technology are still valued and used, but they are at the service of the individual, to be used only when necessary and appropriate and not in a standardised way or as the default option.

Holistic practitioners tend to take a longer-term view, focusing on the creation and maintenance of health and wellbeing, and multiple healing modalities are embraced. In practice, they often question the received knowledge of the technocratic paradigm and seek to 'journey the boundaries' (Wickham 2010). Their goal is not to challenge for the sake of it, but to create and in some cases rediscover some of the knowledge that is lost when we place our sole focus on technology and an objective approach.

Different perspectives within maternity care

All three of these approaches are found within modern maternity care. The technocratic approach is by far the most common, and is the belief system held by many practitioners who work within medical care systems and hospitals. The technocratic approach is also sometimes known as the medical model or the obstetric paradigm and the humanistic and/or holistic approaches correlate somewhat with what we call the midwifery model or social model of care, but there is no direct correlation between someone's role or job and their belief system about birth. Not all doctors are technocratic in their approach; a good few are humanistic and there are some who are more holistic. It is also possible to find midwives and other birth workers who fit into all three of these categories. As health care systems are very technocratic in their approach, it is rather rare (though not impossible) to find truly holistic people working within them. That's because it is quite hard to cope with working in a health care system and having to follow guidelines that go against your basic belief system. There are many humanistic midwives working in health care systems though, and many midwives who work privately or independently are humanistic or holistic in their approach.

As in every walk of life, some people are self-aware about who they are and where they come from in terms of their beliefs, and others might tend to assume that their way is the best or only way without either knowing or thinking about possible alternatives. I don't think anybody who works with birthing women gets up in the morning and thinks, *'Hey, I'm going to disempower a few women today'* or, *'Do you know what? I'm going to go out there and give biased or inaccurate information in order to persuade someone to do what I think is right or best'.* Everyone is doing and advising what they think is best. But it can be good to take a step back in order to work out whose 'best' is most aligned with what you want and believe.

These models aren't fixed, and this is just a simplistic summary of a few patterns which can help form a framework to think about these issues. Many people walk a middle road. Some people find that their views are sometimes conflicting or paradoxical and, as in many areas, there are a whole range of viewpoints rather than just the ones that I've described.

People can change their approach, and the predominant approach within a culture or team or institution can also change over time. Although the technocratic approach currently holds more sway in our culture than some of the other approaches, that doesn't make it more 'right' or true. It's just the approach that reflects the present values of our modern culture, so it could be said to be the current default position. But it wasn't the default position two hundred years ago, and it's highly unlikely to continue to be the default position in the future.

It is my hope that understanding a bit about these belief systems will help you see how these different approaches to birth will shape the experiences of people who are pregnant or giving birth. There's another reason that this information is important, though. If you hold one belief system and you have a primary caregiver who believes something entirely different, then your journey can end up being more difficult than it needs to be. Having a bit of knowledge about different perspectives on childbirth can help prevent that happening.

No matter whether those around you think you can grow, birth and feed your baby easily or think you'll need the help of every test, technology and product available, they'll be looking for what they expect to see. Pregnancy is a very special time, and it is too precious to spend in conflict or uncertainty. For this reason, among many others, it is important to surround yourself with people you can relate to, who respect your outlook on birth and who will truly support your decisions – even if they don't always agree with them – rather than spending your journey feeling that you are in conflict with your travel companion.

But the beliefs that we ourselves hold can also have an enormous impact upon what happens on our pregnancy and birth journeys, so we'll look at that later in the book. Before we move on to that, though, I'm going to look more closely at a really key idea which affects childbirth more than almost any other; the concept of risk.

5. Putting risk into perspective

If it were possible to jump into a time machine and compare the world we live in today with the world as it was in different points in history, we would notice lots of differences. But there's one key and relatively recent feature of our modern world which plays such a huge part in the way we experience pregnancy, childbirth and the decision-making related to this journey (and, frankly, many aspects of the rest of our lives as well) that I think it warrants a chapter of its own. That feature is the idea of risk. Those of us alive today live in a world in which people and companies use the idea of risk to sell products, ideas and suggested behaviour, and that focus plays a huge role in shaping our experiences.

The risk culture

In just a couple of centuries, risk has become a defining feature of our culture and the related emotion fear is used to sell us everything from insurance policies and funeral plans to food, soap and even toothpaste. Potential customers are often told, often subtly but sometimes very loudly, that they are at risk. At the same time, it is implied that the product or service will protect them from or reduce that risk.

And we are built to respond to this. As humans, we are primed to do whatever we can to avoid risk and the possible consequences that we've been led to believe will result from this and so we decide to spend money or take action now in the hope of avoiding some kind of pain or regret later.

I have a friend who lectures in marketing and he has shown me some toe-curling examples of fear-based marketing which he uses to demonstrate how risk and fear are used to create profit. One is an advert for a webcam aimed at parents which raises the question of whether their babysitter is trustworthy. The advert uses some disturbing suggestions and images, along with the marketing message that, if you buy a webcam and monitor from this company, you can watch what your babysitter is up to from the comfort of your candlelit restaurant dinner.

I do wonder if, having been introduced to such disturbing thoughts (which might not otherwise have crossed your mind), you may feel less relaxed during your candlelit dinner after being exposed to such selling tactics. For a start, you've now been introduced to the idea that your babysitter might not take good care of your child so you could be feeling a bit stressed about that. You're also now trying to keep one eye on the screen, which is probably interfering with your levels of oxytocin, the hormone which bonds you and your partner during candlelit dinners (and many other activities) and which is inhibited by stress hormones such as adrenalin. One of you might have decided to forgo a glass of wine so that you can be poised to leap into the car which you felt you needed to bring lest you need to leave quickly in order to rescue your child from the babysitter's impending neglect. Could the level of fear that the company needed to raise in you to persuade you to buy that babysitter monitoring device be having some unintended negative consequences on your evening?

A similar birth-related example is that of electronic monitoring of the heart rates of babies during labour. These machines are marketed on the basis that they help detect when there is a problem, which will allow midwives and doctors to act quickly to get the baby out. But several decades of research have failed to show that having such monitoring leads to better outcomes, and we know that they lead to negative consequences (Sartwelle & Johnston 2015, 2016). One of these, as with the camera example above, is that people actually feel more worried, and thus less relaxed.

Feeling less relaxed is a significant issue when it comes to being in labour, because oxytocin is a key hormone in labour as well as at candlelit dinners. It's part of a complex cocktail of substances which the woman's body releases in order to make labour and birth progress well. The use of monitors and other technology means that women's position and movement is restricted and the fact that their results aren't very accurate means that many women end up having intervention that they don't need. In some situations, the downsides of this kind of interference are outweighed by the potential benefits of the use of technology, but many people argue that their routine use arguably does more harm than good (Sartwelle & Johnston 2015, 2016, Wagner 2000).

There are lots of other examples of this, both in relation to birth and to everyday life. Risk assessment, as I will return to in a bit, tends to carry risks of its own.

Selectively focusing on risk

The use of risk to scare people into spending their money or toeing the line is also pretty selective. So even though our culture is very focused on the notion of risk, it over-focuses on some types of risk while ignoring others completely. Generally, it is used by those who have a technocratic viewpoint and, as a result, it focuses on the things that seem scary or important to those people.

The mass media loves to hype up the alleged risks of home birth (which are not borne out by the research that has been carried out in this area, such as the Birthplace (2011) study). Few to none of the newspaper articles or TV features on this topic ever mention that there are risks attached to giving birth in hospital. Yet all possible birth places, as with any decision that one can make, carry risks or downsides as well as benefits. Hospital birth carries a higher chance of having a caesarean and other interventions than home or birth centre birth and women and babies have a greater chance of developing an infection in hospital than if they stay at home.

There are all sorts of emotional and social consequences as well. Women in hospital are more likely to be separated from their partner and families for at least some of the time and they may not feel able to eat, drink, wear and do what they choose. They may lack privacy, feel lonely, be unable to sleep, feel inhibited, be deprived of their usual nourishment and routines, feel overwhelmed and not receive the same support as they might at home.

That doesn't make it a bad choice, and I'm not trying to put you off it if that's where you want to give birth, but I do want to illustrate how some decisions are widely advertised as being risk-laden, while the risks and downsides of others are never mentioned.

The risks of focusing on risk

Risk-focused marketing is everywhere, and it's not just used by advertisers, but by governments and professionals, either consciously or subconsciously. We have all picked up and use the assumptions and language of our culture and many of us unknowingly transmit these fear-based messages, especially around birth.

Fear is a very powerful tool which can be used subtly or bluntly in order to try and control the decisions that someone makes. It is an effective tool because we humans have inbuilt mechanisms for sniffing out and responding to potential danger. Those mechanisms are really important if you're out there in the woods trying not to get eaten by a bear before you've managed to find a good cave in which to put the kids to bed, but some elements of modern society are causing us to over-focus on it. So many people have become so fear-based in their thinking that they have unwittingly become part of the problem, and I think it's way past time that we had a louder conversation about the way in which the notions of risk and fear are used to try to control people's behaviour and actions in different sectors of our culture.

There's a fine line here though. I am really not trying to make you fearful about fear or risk or those who are using those concepts to sell their ideas, wares, TV programmes or newspapers. I am, however, inviting you to relax your body, still your mind and just to become aware of how these tactics might be affecting you, both in general and in relation to birth.

It might be helpful to think about how fear and risk work

30

together to sell things. In order to sell someone an idea or product through fear, you need to convince them of a few things. You need to convince them that there is an unpleasant outcome which they could experience if they don't do or buy what you say. It is, according to theorists in this area, apparently not enough to highlight an unwanted outcome; you also have to convince the person that they could easily be affected by this outcome and that they have the ability to make a decision which would enable them to avoid the pain. These things don't necessarily have to be true; in fact they often are not true. I'm just saying that's what you need to do if you want to use the notions of risk and fear to sell an idea, product or service.

The good news is that we do have some control over the extent to which we embrace the modern notion of risk and allow it to affect our lives. Awareness of this issue is not just the first step but actually the biggest step that anyone can take towards removing themselves from the grip of fear-based persuasion. Once someone has seen that this particular emperor isn't wearing any clothes (so to speak), their awareness of that is always there, and they are more able to make decisions based on what's right for them rather than what's right for or what's believed by the person trying to sell their approach.

Risk and birth

Whether they intend to or not, both lay and professional people frequently imply that certain pregnancy and birth-related decisions are safer or riskier than others. So fear is used to promote particular birth interventions and approaches. As we have seen, these statements are often either not true or only part of the picture. But even untrue or partially true statements have the effect of introducing fear into the conversation. People may find themselves concerned about their or their baby's wellbeing, questioning their decisions and wondering whether they should choose something else, whether that is an actual product or a different service, intervention or idea. In many cases, we have so fully absorbed the idea (often in our childhood) that certain birth-related decisions are risk-laden that we wouldn't dream of considering another option. But if you read the research evidence that looks at these areas or talk to people who have experienced the reality of various experiences, the truth is often very different from the hype.

Some maternity care systems and birth practitioners categorise women as either 'low risk' (or healthy, which is a far more positive way of saying the same thing) or 'high risk'. But it's important to understand a couple of things about these labels.

Firstly, you don't have to accept being labelled with a risk status at all. You may have noticed that there is no category of 'no risk' within modern maternity services. That's partly because the technocratic paradigm is very focused on risk. And if you place your focus on looking for risk then you'll soon realise that things can always go awry, even if the chance of that happening is one in a trillion. Even spending your day wrapped up in cotton wool and safely locked in a bank vault guarded by dragons doesn't rule out the possibility that something untoward could happen. In fact, adding the cotton wool, locks and dragons might even increase the chance of a problem.

This is the journey of life. By its very nature, life is filled with uncertainty and surprise. We might not be able to change the fact that our culture is filled with notions of fear and risk. But we don't have to accept being labelled as 'at risk' and let it ruin our day.

Secondly, the rather worrying category of 'high risk', which makes it sound as if women are walking around just waiting for a disaster to occur, doesn't mean what many people think it does. In most cases, it means that a woman has a marginally to slightly higher chance of experiencing a problem than the women who have no known problems and who have been labelled as 'low risk'. It's still really unlikely that a 'high risk' woman will ever experience that problem, and I'll explain more on the numbers of this in the very next section, and there are almost certainly things she can do to increase her chance of not having that problem.

Carrie, when told that she was at 'high risk', decided to go and read the statistics for herself. When she discovered that the actual risk was much lower than she had feared, she chose to focus on the positive things she could do to improve her and her baby's health, which included improving her nutrition, joining a pregnancy yoga class and seeking a therapist who could help her to de-stress. It's often a matter of deciding what perspective you are going to take.

Absolute and relative risk

There is one very important final thing that I'd like to share while I'm on the subject of risk. I'd like to explain the concepts of absolute and relative risk, because I think that these are well worth knowing about if you are doing anything (like considering or experiencing pregnancy and birth) which is going to involve people telling you about the risks of different paths that one might take.

People are often worried into action when they hear that their chances of a problem will be doubled or trebled (or halved or quartered) if they do or do not take a particular course of action, such as having their labour induced or declining a test or intervention. That's partly because, when we hear that something is several times more or less likely, it triggers us into thinking that there is a big difference and that something is much more dangerous or risky than what it is being compared to. These comparative figures – halved, doubled, seventeen times more likely - is what we mean when we talk about relative risk: we are discussing the risk of something relative to the risk of something else.

But relative risk can be confusing and misleading, and not only because some people find numbers hard to understand. Firstly, when some people hear that the chance of something has doubled, they think they have a 50/50 chance of experiencing it, and that's not the case at all. It is, in fact, impossible to know the extent to which the chance of something has changed unless you also know the numbers relating to the absolute risk or the actual chance of something happening.

Let's take a really unrelated example. Please imagine that you are considering buying a new toy for your excitable new puppy. Your puppy eats everything and so you want to know whether there is a risk that, if he chews the paint off his new toy, he will become ill. *"Well"*, says the puppy toy salesperson. *"There is a risk, yes. So if you buy this other toy instead, which is three times the price, the risk is halved and your dog is safer."*

Whether or not you will be swayed towards buying the more expensive toy will depend on a number of factors. But if you know about absolute and relative risk then you'll want to ask the salesperson for one more piece of information: what is the actual or absolute risk of a problem with each toy.

"Well", says the dog toy salesperson again. *"Studies have found that the risk of a problem with the cheaper toy is one in a million. But that is halved with the more expensive toy, and the risk is one in two million."*

If everything else was equal, which would you buy?

I hope this illustrates the issue, and the reason why I am saying that it is important to know the absolute risk as well as the relative risk. There are other things we could ask as well, of course. I haven't spent time looking at risk and dogs, but I would bet that there are other things that would pose a far higher threat to your imaginary new puppy than eating paint from toys. If, as a diligent dog lover, you spotted early signs of paint chewing and removed the toy, would that solve the problem? And it doesn't hurt to dig even deeper and ask about the source of the information that you're being offered, but I'll have more to say about that in chapter 7.

Let's look at some absolute and relative risk examples from maternity care. Firstly, to put all of this into context, I'd like to tell you that the crude perinatal mortality rate in the UK in a report published in 2016 was 5.92 in 1000 (MBRRACE-UK 2016). That is, one in 169 babies. It's sad to think about and there are lots of different reasons for that, and of course we want to do what we can to change that. We know that this doesn't always mean doing more, however, because interventions carry risks of their own and can sometimes do more harm than good. I want you to have that overall figure to bear in mind, because that will enable you to put some of the figures that I am about to share into context.

My first example concerns babies who are in a breech position at the end of pregnancy, which means their mothers need to decide whether to have a vaginal birth or a caesarean section. There are pros and cons to each, as with most things.

An obstetrician friend of mine teaches students about absolute and relative risk by having them look at the statistics which relate to giving birth to a breech baby either vaginally or by caesarean section. Different research studies give slightly different figures on this, but the paper she uses to illustrate this is a meta-analysis (Berhan & Haileamlak 2015) which gathers together data from lots of different studies.

If you take the results of this analysis and look at the relative risk of perinatal death in vaginal breech birth compared to caesarean section, you would find out that the risk of death is seven times higher in vaginal birth than caesarean section, which sounds like a lot. But the absolute risk of perinatal death for breech babies born vaginally is 0.35%, which is 3.5 in 1000, or 1 in 286 babies. When students (and women) look at the absolute risk in this area, they often feel rather differently about the risks and benefits of the two options, especially as caesarean section carries a number of risks for the mother and baby which vaginal birth does not.

Another topical example is found in the trend towards offering older women induction of labour, simply because they are older. We do not yet have any good data to show that induction of labour makes a difference in this scenario, and one commonly cited paper on this topic (RCOG 2013) shows how the relative and absolute risk relate to each other. As the paper shows, the relative risk of stillbirth in an older woman is almost twice that of a younger woman, but even at 41 weeks of pregnancy the absolute risk of stillbirth (including babies who have medical problems) for a woman who is 40 years old is 1 in 463. And again, there are other risks from induction of labour, so the decision needs to be made by the individual woman. The overall point is that, when you look closely at the numbers, the difference and the decision isn't always quite as cut and dried as the relative risk statistics might have made you think it is.

Don't be too surprised, however, if the person telling you doesn't actually know what the numbers are themselves. When I am teaching research and statistics, I find that people often remember the relative risk far better than they remember absolute numbers. But if the person you're talking to is a care provider or someone whose job it is to know this stuff, then do ask them to get you the information so that you can make an informed decision. Although some people make the difference between different decisions sound vast, the actual increase in risk is often no different to the risk of driving your car to the shops when it's drizzling with rain as opposed to driving it to the same shops on a sunny day. And a bit of rain doesn't usually stop people from going where they want to go!

6. Considering your own beliefs about life, birth and information

Now that we've looked at some of the bigger issues about the things that affect birth decisions, I'm going to move on to some practical suggestions and tools. Some people find it valuable to spend a bit of time pondering their current beliefs and knowledge about pregnancy, birth and parenting. That's what this chapter offers.

This activity doesn't need to involve in-depth analysis with a therapist (unless you want it to), but reflecting on your experiences, knowledge, beliefs and feelings can sometimes highlight what you need or want in pregnancy and birth. It can also help you decide where you stand, and perhaps which of the paradigms described in chapter 4 you feel most aligned with. Once you know that, you can then focus on finding the kind of care, practitioner and setting that will be right for you.

Below are lots of questions that might help you think through your own philosophy and the sources of your beliefs about birth. You might want to read these questions just as you're reading the rest of the book and trust that, if something is important, it will jump off the page at you. Another option is to read this section more slowly, or plan to come back to it later. Or you might want to use the questions as an exercise, in which case you can either think through the questions alone or sit with someone else and have them ask you the questions as if they were interviewing you. If you have a partner, you may want to discuss these questions with them, perhaps having read or worked through them together or separately, as they may lead to useful insights about the way you both feel. Or maybe there's someone else you feel it would be useful to talk this through with.

As with all of these ideas, there's no right or wrong, and nobody is trying to change your mind. There are more than 60 questions in this chapter, and of course you don't need to answer all of them. This is simply an invitation to consider your existing beliefs (and maybe also to think about how you feel about what you have read so far) so that you can decide whether they really are yours or whether any of them are other people's ideas that don't serve you or your family.

What were your childhood experiences of pregnancy and birth? What did your mother and other relatives tell you about birth, or about your own birth?

Whether you are aware of it or not, the knowledge you gained about birth as a child may impact on the way you feel about birth now. As children, we sometimes hear and internalise other people's beliefs without really being aware of it. Are these acquired beliefs serving you well today?

Have you ever attended any births? If so, how did they affect you?

Bear in mind that seeing one or two labours or births may not mean you have a representative image of birth in general. What did you learn from the births you attended? Would you like to experience that kind of birth? If not, what would you change?

Can you recall any pregnancy or birth stories from TV shows, films or other media sources that have stuck in your mind?

I often tell couples in birth preparation sessions that the only place I wouldn't recommend having their baby is in a soap opera. That's because people who give birth in soap operas have a very high chance of having their baby somewhere other than where they intended, and the rate of unexpected complications is incredibly high. If they don't have an unintended medical complication, they are likely to end up having their baby either in a broken-down van on the side of the road (with a farm hand as an impromptu midwife), or prematurely and in a stable surrounded by live donkeys.

The latter is great for ratings, because it means that the birth scene will make a lovely final tableau for the Christmas Day episode. It is not, unfortunately, so great for the viewers, who may end up unconsciously absorbing the ideas that birth is dangerous and that most labours last for less than half an hour. Also, many of the babies born on TV don't have umbilical cords, the placenta never gets a mention and the babies themselves tend to be a few days or weeks old at birth.

The problem of this high-peril, high-drama approach is that these made-up, unrealistic stories tend to stay with us and form some of our ideas about what birth is like. This problem has been made worse by some of the reality TV shows which depict birth, as these often focus on women who are experiencing unusual situations.

Do you think that you might have picked up unrealistic, overly dramatic or high-peril ideas about birth from TV, films or the internet? If so, is there a chance that these have coloured your own viewpoint and made you feel more stressed than is warranted?

What have your friends told you about their births? What birth stories have you read or heard elsewhere?

Listening to positive birth stories can be a wonderful thing for a pregnant woman and those who will be with her during labour and birth. Unfortunately, there are also many scary or negative birth stories out there, and hearing these is not always helpful for pregnant women.

It's important to understand that there's a bigger picture here, though. People who have had a distressing time sometimes need to tell and retell their stories many times, in order to process their experiences. Some of these people go on to campaign for tests, interventions or features of care that they think (not always correctly) may have made a difference to their own experience. They may not realise that their words and actions can make other people feel distressed or disempowered.

But other people have realised that this negative bias can exist and have gone out of their way to make positive birth stories available. A great example of this is the website http://tellmeagoodbirthstory.com/

Thinking back over the birth stories that you have heard, can you recall any particularly positive or negative birth stories? Do any feel neutral? How have you been affected by stories that you have heard, and how do you feel about this?

What are your fundamental beliefs about birth? Can you identify where these beliefs come from?

Having now looked at a few of these questions and considered how other people and viewpoints might have influenced you, how do you feel right now? If you are surprised by the way you feel about childbirth in general or one aspect of it in particular, you might like to spend some time reflecting on why you might feel this way. Can you identify possible influences upon your current viewpoint from your previous experiences?

Do you like, dislike, trust or fear your body? How do you feel about your body?

Our self-image is shaped by opinions from many sources, including family, friends, society and the media. Do you feel positive about your body and gender? Do you feel negative? How do you feel about your menstrual cycle? About menopause, birth, aging? About the shape of your body?

How do you feel about the judgements that our culture makes about the way that you look or the size you are? What about the things that some people feel a woman should do (like shaving or waxing, trimming or removing some or all of their pubic and armpit hair, putting on make-up, wearing high heels and so on) in order to be perceived as acceptable and/or desirable?

Do any of your feelings surprise you?

Do you feel that these feelings and views are your own, or have any of them come from elsewhere? Are they viewpoints that you agree with?

How do you want your baby to feel about their body? Are there things that you might want to read, consider or do in order to maximise the chance of your baby picking up positive messages from you?

What do you feel women need from their birth experience?

If you were making a list of the basic physical, social, emotional and spiritual needs of women who are giving birth, what would you put on it? What attributes do you think somebody who looks after women in labour should have? What else should be available? What do you feel women should be able to expect from their birth and birth attendant?

Once you have made these lists, you might like to consider which of the needs you have listed are related to the environment, which could be met by other people and which need to be met by the caregiver who will attend the birth?

But let's return to the birthing environment. What kind of environment do you think you would like to give birth in? Could you describe your ideal birth environment? My aim in asking this question is to get you to think about what you need first and then consider what's actually available and out there. That's because I think it's much better to be able to look for a setting and caregiver who fits what you and your family need and want rather than feeling that you need to mould yourself to what is on offer from the first person or care setting that you find.

What did you feel about your previous birth or health experiences?

Again, previous experience can impact our future decisions. If you have had a previous pregnancy or given birth before, what was this experience like and how did you feel about it? Did you enjoy your previous pregnancies and births? Are there things you wish had happened differently?

If this raises issues for you, do you need to talk these through with someone who might be able to explain things you don't understand or help you make sense of them? If so, and you are still living in the same area, you may be able to meet with the person who cared for you or a local birth debriefing service to talk through what happened. Do follow your instincts with this, though. If you didn't have a good experience, it may not be helpful to meet with the person or someone representing the place who cared for you. And while some birth debriefing services are genuinely woman-centred, I am aware that in some cases women have felt that the people they met were focused more on defending and justifying what happened rather than on helping the woman to work through her own feelings about her experience.

If you haven't been pregnant or given birth before, think about previous health experiences instead, for example your experiences with therapists, doctors, dentists or a school nurse. How would you describe these experiences? How do you feel about them? Are there things that you wish had happened differently? Do you have positive memories of a caregiver that might help you work out what you want from someone who will be with you in labour?

Do you have other life experiences which could impact on your experience of pregnancy or birth?

These might be positive experiences that could help you think about what you want from your birth, or they might be negative experiences. Sadly, many women have been (or are being) sexually, physically or emotionally abused, and many others have mental health problems or find themselves in other difficult situations. Such experiences or situations may cause you to feel you need a particular type of care or caregiver, or you may be feeling that there are particular settings, situations or procedures that you need or want to avoid. If you are in this situation, it can really help if you can find someone who you can talk to and who will help you communicate your needs. This might be your midwife or doctor, but if you do not feel that you can talk to them straight away, then perhaps a friend, doula or someone else who you see professionally may be able to help or support you.

What sources of knowledge do you value the most?

At this point in time, our society generally values scientific, rational knowledge above other types of knowledge, although if you talk to people who study philosophy or social sciences, they will tell you that there is a large question mark over whether any knowledge can really be objective and rational. But there are lots of other types of knowledge and sources of information, and different people and families and cultures value these in different ways. Some examples of information sources include knowledge from scientific research, other people's stories, the opinions of midwives, doctors or other professionals, knowledge of bodily physiology, knowledge from practitioners with a non-technocratic approach, other women's life experiences, your own intuition or inner knowledge, spiritual insights and common sense reasoning.

Which of those kinds of knowledge do you value? Which do your partner, family or friends value?

Women and their families are offered lots of different types of information during pregnancy and birth and they often find that they need to filter it in order to decide what is right for them. All forms of knowledge can be useful, but all can also be misleading if we don't think about them critically. It can be useful to take a step back from a particular piece of information and to consider whether it is truly something that you want to take on board in your decision making.

Do you think that your views on knowledge and information are aligned with, or different from, those of your loved ones, partner, family, friends, caregiver and/or the society or culture that you live in?

In one sense, it doesn't matter whether anyone else agrees with your viewpoint or not. It is your viewpoint and you are entitled to hold it, live by it and make your decisions by it. But if there are fundamental birth-related things about which you and your partner or family disagree, then it may be better to uncover and discuss these earlier rather than later.

If there are fundamental things on which you and your caregiver disagree, then it may be time to consider looking for a different caregiver. (See appendix 2 for information on this). This is your pregnancy and birth. You are at the centre of this experience, and you do not need to bend to anyone else's view. I have said this before, but it is important to surround yourself with people who will respect your wishes in labour but also let you know if circumstances change and a different path may be advisable. You may find that you are less able to advocate for yourself in labour, especially once your hormones start to do their thing. Women often find that they need to reach deep inside themselves, and it is really important to know that whoever is with you will protect you and allow you to switch off from what is happening around you, knowing that your viewpoint is heard, understood and respected.

How do you feel about body knowledge and intuition?

I write a lot about people's own knowledge about their bodies and the concept of intuition, because I value these things a lot. That's partly because, as a midwife, I have seen time and time again how valuable women's knowledge can be. Women know things about their bodies and their babies that we just can't find out through technology or science, so we need to learn to listen to women.

To what extent do you trust, follow and make decisions by the sensations that you experience in your body, or by insights that come to you? What do you feel about bodily and intuitive knowledge generally? Is this something that you would like to consider or explore further?

What are your hopes and goals? What are your fears? What do you feel most strongly about? What questions do you have?

Pondering these questions can help you determine what your priorities are for this pregnancy and birth. Even if you think you know this already, it may still be worth asking yourself these questions as you may be surprised by some of the answers. If you find that you were aware of the answers to all of these questions, you can be pleased that you are so in tune with your desires.

Are there any other aspects of your life experience or current situation that you feel might be important in influencing the way you feel about your birth?

Look back over any notes you might have made so far. Can you think of anything else that might act as an influence or affect the way you feel? Do you have a clearer sense about what your feelings, priorities, hopes and concerns are?

Are there issues that you feel you need to talk through more with someone else? Who could you ask for help?

What can you learn from comparing notes with your partner? Have you considered or written any answers which have surprised you, or uncovered things that you didn't realise were important? What have you gained from this exercise, and are there things you want to look into, change or reconsider as a result of doing this?

What are three things you learned from this?

Sometimes, people make lots of notes when they do this exercise, and are then not sure where to go with it. That's what this last question is about. No matter whether you read this chapter, spend time writing or discussing it or approached it in any other way, here's one last question to consider before you move on. What are three things you learned from doing this, or from your reading of the book so far? Sometimes, it's helpful to crystallise thinking by trying to come up with a small number of take-home messages, so I'm inviting you to consider what yours are before you move on to the next chapter which looks more generally at information and offers tips for weighing it up.

7. A few tips on weighing up information

The journey through pregnancy, birth and parenting brings with it the need to consider information from a number of sources. When someone becomes pregnant, they are almost instantly bombarded with leaflets, books, offers of 'helpful' (but often unsolicited) advice and the veritable flood of birth-related information on the internet.

We all know that the quality and accuracy of information can be very variable, and that it can be important to think about where information has come from and how valid it is, but it's not always easy to work out how to differentiate between information which comes from alternative sources. This chapter offers a few general thoughts about weighing up birth-related information, and in the next chapters I will look at specific kinds of birth-related decisions in more depth.

It can be helpful to understand that people share information in a variety of ways. Some people focus on offering the information and decision in as objective a way as they can and get you to do all the deciding. Some offer reassurance and more of a 'guide on the side' approach, where they try and establish what you want, offer the information that you need and then work out how to actively support you on your journey. Others feel that they already know what the best path is for you. That might be because they feel they know you well, they have found that something works for others, they think everybody should do the same, they feel that other paths are scary or they just have an 'I know best' approach. You might also encounter people who simply expect that you will do as you are told. Trust your intuition, 'spidey sense' or gut feeling about this stuff. When you first encounter information, be curious about how it has been gathered, how it is presented and whether it might be biased.

Bias is everywhere, but it isn't always easy to spot. Most people already realise that, if they are reading an information leaflet which has been sponsored by a company which makes a particular product, it may be a fair assumption that the information will be designed to make you feel you should buy or have that product, rather than being balanced in outlining the advantages and disadvantages of the product. But sometimes, the small print is very small and hard to spot. Sometimes it's not there at all. Such information can also be subtly biased and there are some grey areas as well.

Some voluntary organisations, for example, might be more able to give unbiased information than a help line sponsored by a company that is seeking to make a profit, but there also exist charities and voluntary organisations that are either very commercially-focused or very biased in their goals. Most commonly, the latter situation is found where people have formed a charity because they weren't given a particular test or intervention or piece of advice in their own birth experience and they are campaigning to ensure that other women get this. Others focus on a rare but harmful disease or condition. Unfortunately, although these people may be very well-intentioned, the advice, test or intervention might not be what other women want or need, it might not be effective or it may carry risks that don't outweigh the benefits for everyone. The people who are campaigning have often been very affected by their own experiences, and can sometimes take a 'we know what's best for you and your baby' approach. These campaigns often use emotive pictures and stories, as it is known that these are good ways of persuading people to take a particular course of action. That's not always fair to those who are subject to them, but you can protect yourself a bit by being aware that this happens.

Finding a path through the information jungle

I am aware that, when it comes to trying to make your way through information, it can sometimes feel like you're trying to make your way through a jungle. I hope that the following list of questions and examples might help you to make a decision when you are faced with a source of information, whether this is a person, a leaflet, a book, a website, a social media post or some other source of information.

Who has produced / paid for this information to be produced and distributed?

Are they impartial, or might they have a vested interest in you making a particular choice? An infant formula company is unlikely to be the best source of breastfeeding information, and a charity selling baby products might not be quite as parent-centred and unbiased as they would like you to think they are. Some or all of their information might still be useful but, as with all of these examples, it is good to consider it within the context of their own aims, which will help you decide whether it is useful for you.

Does this information / source discuss just one option, or a range of options?

Realistically, the way in which we specialise in our work means that it's hard to get everything you need from one source. You are unlikely, for instance, to get detailed information about the differences between spinal and epidural anaesthesia from a homeopath and neither will an anaesthetist be an expert on all of the non-pharmacological things that can be used to alleviate discomfort or pain.

In another example, mainstream health services are not

likely to offer information about private or independent midwives or birth centres, and they may also not tell you about doula services which you might want to access in addition to mainstream care. So be aware of the area of expertise that is covered by a source of information. Are you happy with the breadth of information that you have, or do you want to look for more? Luckily, it's relatively easy to cast your net more widely using the internet, especially if you're prepared to step outside your comfort zone and look around a bit. Appendix 1 offers lots of suggestions as to how you can find out more and the kinds of people and groups you might want to look for.

What does the person who is giving me this information really believe about birth?

I've covered what this means and why it might be important in chapter 4. In order to find this out, you can either ask them directly about their philosophy and beliefs, or come up with some key questions which will help you figure out where they might be coming from. Good questions include, *"how many of the women you look after end up having a spontaneous labour and a straightforward vaginal birth without intervention?"* or *"what is your feeling about pain relief in labour?"*

The answers to both of those questions should give you a bit of a clue about what their underpinning values are. If they are unwilling to discuss these things, or if they make a joke of the question or gloss over the issues, that should set off warning bells. If you have any say in the matter, you may want to keep looking for someone who will take your questions seriously. If you don't feel that you can change your caregiver for whatever reason, then you may want to get people around you who will advocate for you and support your decisions.

What is the original source of this information?

Do remember that it is a very human thing to spin information, and it is not necessarily done knowingly or on purpose. It's also common for people to remember and retell only part of the information that they encounter. So it's very reasonable and useful to ask people (or books, or websites, and we'll come back to that in the next point) where they got their information from.

Practitioners who are unwilling to discuss the source of their information with you may not be open to sharing decision-making with you, especially in more intense circumstances, such as during labour. A good question here is, *"that's interesting … I would like to think about that. Would you be able to provide me with the evidence, so I can look into it more deeply myself?"*

Is the source of this information verifiable?

Be particularly wary of information that comes from journalistic sources via television, newspapers and the internet. Google is a great tool to get quick answers to things, but the answers may not always serve you well. The creators of the information may be more interested in a story, spin, scandal or product promotion than in offering fair and unbiased information to their audience.

Be particularly wary of clickbait, and of sites that are full of advertising. Both search engine experts and ad-heavy website owners are well aware of the key things that expecting parents are worrying about and likely to type into a search engine. Search engines are paid by baby product, pharmaceutical and technology companies to send people to their sites.

Even magazines which deal specifically in parenting and birth issues may not be offering information based on anything more than the opinion of the writer and they often only present a very mainstream view. If they present more than one viewpoint, these will often be the extremes of the possibilities, whereas most women will find that their experience is not that extreme.

Websites run by professional organisations are a good source of information on what the standard advice on something is, but they are generally conservative and may be more aligned with a technocratic perspective. However, you'll also find websites offering what appears to be very holistic, woman-centred information and yet, on closer inspection, you'll find that it is all theory and not backed up by good evidence or experience. If the website or blog is run by a professional, read their 'About' page to find out about who they are and what they have to say for themselves and also see whether they are directly promoting a product or service to women and families.

Finally, ask yourself, does this information feel right? Does it fit well with your own beliefs and philosophy?

If you have a nagging feeling of doubt about something you have been told, even if it comes from a seemingly trustworthy source, I would encourage you to trust that feeling and focus on finding out more. Or, if you feel really drawn to something that you might not otherwise have considered or tried, pay attention to that too. Your intuitive mind might be trying to tell you something which your rational brain has missed.

8. Understanding birth intervention: four types of intervention

Many of the decisions that women and families need to make during the childbearing year are to do with the different interventions offered by birth attendants and facilities. The range of interventions used in pregnancy and childbirth is vast, and each intervention brings possible advantages and possible risks and side effects. The task of making decisions about which interventions (if any) will be right for you and your baby can seem enormous, no matter whether these are things that are offered routinely or whether you are told that you have a higher than average chance of having a problem.

Different interventions are offered for different reasons and purposes, and knowing what kind of intervention you're being offered and what its purpose is can help you to ask the right questions and get the information that you need to make a decision about it. In the moment, however, there may not be time to learn about all that, even if the person in front of you is aware that it might be helpful – and often they may not be.

When I wrote the very first version of this book, back in 2002, I realised that it might be useful to put birth interventions into simplified categories and then share a few basic things about each category with women and their families, with the most important thing being the questions that they might want to ask when considering whether a particular intervention is right for them.

Hundreds of women and men have since told me that this was one of the most useful things I ever did for them, because it made decision-making less daunting by giving them a bit of background knowledge and a framework to use even when they felt that they were otherwise alone. I have developed these ideas even more since then, and this chapter goes through the four different types of intervention and the kind of questions that you might want to ask of each of them.

Please don't forget that you are entitled to equally respectful and non-judgmental treatment whether you decide to accept or decline tests or interventions.

The four types of intervention

The four different types of intervention which are offered to women and babies during pregnancy, labour, birth and the postnatal and neonatal periods are:

Screening tests
Clinical interventions
Prophylactic interventions
Elective interventions

Each of these types of intervention is offered for a slightly different reason. Because of this, there are specific questions which can be asked about each which will help you gain the information you need to help you make decisions about whether they are right for you and your baby. There's some overlap between a couple of these but I have spelled the list out twice, because I know that people use this as a quick reference guide. So no apology for a bit of repetition here!

I'll go through each of these types of intervention in turn over the next few pages. I'll outline the reasoning behind each, let you know what the wider issues are and suggest some questions you could ask when gathering information on them from your birth attendant and other sources.

Screening tests

Screening tests are the most common intervention offered to childbearing women. I use the term 'offered' loosely, because some are seen as such an everyday and normal part of pregnancy that many caregivers and women just assume will routinely happen, and don't even think to question them.

Examples of screening tests include blood pressure checks, checking a woman's urine, measuring her height and weight to calculate BMI, ultrasound examination, vaginal examination, blood testing on the woman or baby, electronic fetal monitoring and most of what happens in an antenatal or postnatal check.

Some screening tests are offered to all women or babies. Others, such as screening for gestational diabetes or swabbing to see if a woman is carrying the Group B Strep bacteria, are offered only to some people. Whether or not you are offered a screening test can sometimes depend on where you live, who is caring for you and whether they perceive that you or your baby are at risk of having or developing a particular disease, complication or problem.

Screening tests are used in order to try to detect deviations from normal. Quite often, especially in pregnancy and labour, screening tests appear to be interventions that are carried out on the woman, but they are actually screening the baby. A good example of this is where a midwife or doctor feels (palpates) the woman's abdomen during pregnancy. Among other things, they are determining whether the baby is growing as expected or whether there are concerns that might warrant further discussion or exploration.

You may already have realised that a big issue when it comes to screening tests relates to the question of who defines what is normal. If the definition of what is normal is widened or narrowed, then that can change things a lot. This is a big issue within maternity care and something that often gets discussed when I am teaching a group of midwives and doctors who work in different areas of the world, because practitioners and systems have different definitions and comfort zones when it comes to defining normality.

There are also quite a few areas where the generally accepted definition of normal is not supported by good evidence, or where there is significant debate and disagreement between different groups of people. One of these is the area of so-called 'post-term' pregnancy, and women in different parts of the world (or in some cases different parts of the same country) will be told different things about this. The same woman would be offered induction at different times depending on where she is in the world, and sometimes where she is in the same country.

Other examples include screening and treatment for women whose babies may be at risk from Group B Strep disease, which also varies geographically (see Wickham 2019) and gestational diabetes, where the cut off points used to decide who has this varies considerably between different areas. This can be really unhelpful for women. It is partly a consequence of there being different perspectives on birth (which I described in chapter 4) but it again illustrates how information isn't as objective as we might like to think.

There is another issue which is important to consider when you are deciding whether to have a screening test. If something is found to be outside of so-called normal limits, can anything be done about this? This is a really vital question because there are situations where, even if a problem or abnormality is detected, there is little or nothing that can be done to help or correct this. But knowing that something is deemed to be unusual or not quite as expected can lead to unnecessary worry.

It is always good to ask and think about the consequences of a screening test. In some situations, for instance, a woman who is found to be outside normal limits will be told that a particular option (such as giving birth at the local birth centre) is no longer available to her, so there are more consequences of having a screening test than you might realise. A good example of this is where women are tested to see if they are carrying Group B Strep bacteria. If this is found to be the case then they may find they are told that they are no longer eligible to give birth in a midwifery-led unit or birth centre (see Group B Strep Explained (Wickham 2019) for more) and they may be put under pressure to accept intravenous antibiotics during labour.

Questions to consider with screening tests

What will the test involve, and what are the benefits and downsides?

Why are you being offered this test? Is the test invasive, painful, expensive, time-consuming? Does it carry a risk to the woman or baby? What could the psychological impact of the test be? (Many women find that waiting for the results of tests, particularly for screening tests that are offered during pregnancy, can be very stressful.) Is the outcome of the screening test going to affect your care and/or the decisions you can make? Will it limit your options in any way?

What information will you receive, and how accurate is the test?

With all screening tests, there is a margin of error and a number of people will get false results. This includes being told that all is well when actually it is not (a false negative) and being told that there is a problem when this is not the case (a false positive). The results of tests are not always clear-cut and you may have to make decisions based on possibilities (or probabilities, if we use the correct mathematical term) rather than on certainties. Sometimes, different areas or professionals will use different cut-off points, which further illustrates that knowledge is not fixed.

If the test highlights something outside of what are considered normal limits, is there anything that can be done about this?

Sometimes there isn't anything we can do to change something, so it's then important to think about whether you would actually want to know if you or your baby had a problem. You may also wish to consider whether what you would be offered would be acceptable to you.

For instance, if you consented to a vaginal examination during labour and the person who performed it felt the results showed that you had not made satisfactory progress, would you consent to being given drugs in an attempt to speed up your labour?

Clinical interventions

I use the term clinical interventions to describe the tools and technologies, drugs and other interventions which are used in an attempt to bring a situation back in line with what are considered to be the normal limits of pregnancy, labour, birth or the postnatal period.

Clinical interventions are often suggested (as in the example of speeding up labour if someone feels it isn't progressing quickly enough) where a screening test has shown that something has moved outside of the so-called normal limits. As I often point out to midwives, doulas and other birth workers in my workshops, this category can also include non-medical interventions such as the use of herbs, essential oils or rebozos (large shawls which some midwives and birth workers use to assist women to make rhythmic movements and get into beneficial positions) or physical positioning or manipulation, depending on what the aim or intention in using them is.

To continue with the example of slow labour progress, the Western medical clinical intervention that might follow the use of vaginal examination as a screening test to determine whether labour was progressing well would be an intravenous drip containing a drug which might speed up labour. Midwives and others who work in out-of-hospital settings also use a range of low-tech alternatives to try to achieve the same end, but these alternatives may or may not be seen as acceptable in a hospital. Examples include suggesting certain kinds of movement (e.g. walking or trying different positions or types of furniture), activity (e.g. kissing or nipple stimulation or using a birth pool or footbath) or manipulations (perhaps with the aid of a rebozo). But it's also worth knowing that many humanistic and holistic midwives and practitioners feel (and know from research evidence) that it's really OK for labour to take longer in some women, as long as mother and baby are coping.

Clinical interventions should be used on an individual basis, so in response to the needs of the individual woman rather than as a routine part of care. However, some systems of care recommend clinical interventions routinely, such as inducing all women's labours at a certain stage of pregnancy, because a woman is older or her pregnancy was conceived through IVF or other reproductive technology.

Other examples of clinical intervention which are more medical in nature include iron or blood transfusion and instrumental or operative delivery. Many of the drugs that are given in pregnancy and childbirth are given because something (such as the woman's blood pressure or the baby's temperature) is perceived to be outside of normal limits.

All of this also returns us to the questions about how we define normal, and who defines that. Do your ideas of normality agree with those of your attendant or facility? This is more likely to be the case if you share the same general approach as your caregivers, as discussed in chapter 4. And, because the recommendation for a clinical intervention may be based on the results of a screening test, you might also want to consider or ask about the accuracy of the screening test on which the suggestion for this intervention was based.

Decisions need to be based on an understanding of what is likely to happen if things are left to continue versus what is likely to happen if you consent to the treatment, drug or intervention that you are being offered. Sometimes, there is more than one alternative that you might want to consider.

Questions to consider with clinical interventions

Many people use the BRAN/BRAIN/BRAINS acronym in this situation (Wickham 2017), and this can be helpful as a reminder of the questions you might want to ask in such a situation. BRAINS stands for:

What are the Benefits?

What are your caregivers hoping will happen if you agree to this intervention? Does the intervention usually work? For what proportion of women or babies does it work? Is the answer to that last question based on evidence or experience?

What are the Risks?

What are the physical and psychological side effects of this intervention? Are there other downsides/ implications? What are your chances of experiencing these? Is there a possibility that this intervention will lead to a 'cascade of intervention'? By 'cascade of intervention', we mean the situation where one intervention tends to lead to another and/or causes a level of discomfort which leads to a woman needing pain relief which limits her movement and has other effects which ultimately lead to her needing a caesarean or instrumental birth.

What are the Alternatives?

Are there other (perhaps less invasive) things that you can try first? If you are being offered a drug, there will often be a herbal or other alternative, although a medical doctor or a midwife employed by a health system may not know or be able to tell you about these.

If you are being offered something to speed up labour, walking around (or even cuddling and kissing with your partner) may achieve the same thing. Water baths or showers and massage are alternatives to narcotic analgesia. If you need pharmaceutical drugs, there is often more than one option here too. You may, for instance, want to look at the risks and benefits of each option or the implications for breastfeeding.

What does my Intuition tell me?

Again, this is about tapping into your gut feeling, body knowledge or sense of what is happening in your pregnancy or labour (or wherever you are on your journey). Remember that your own knowledge is just as valid as other forms of knowledge and it may tell you more in certain situations.

What if I do Nothing?

What are the possible scenarios or consequences if I do not agree to this intervention, and how likely is each of these? Can we wait a while and see what happens before I make a decision about this? Doing nothing doesn't necessarily mean you're deciding to never act or do something. While doing nothing can mean saying an absolute no, it can instead mean deciding to do nothing for now and waiting for another ten minutes or an hour or a day before reconsidering your decision. In other words, there is a difference between 'deciding to decline' and 'deciding to wait and see'.

Smile, 'Scuse yourself or ask for a Second opinion?

The 's' of BRAINS can reminds us of a few different things, depending on who you hear it from. These include a reminder that we may be more likely to get helpful answers by asking such questions with a smile. While a part of me thinks that we should be able to get helpful answers without having to do extra work to ease the communication ourselves, the reality is that the default viewpoint in our culture is the risk-focused, medical one and it can sometimes take a bit of extra effort to get non-standard information from people working within systems that often constrain what they feel they can say. For example, clinical guidelines used by healthcare professionals to assist decision making can be mistakenly viewed (and used) as policies to 'enforce' decision making.

For other educators, the 's' is a good reminder that you can say 'scuse me' and tell people you need time to think and that you also have a right to a second opinion.

Prophylactic interventions

Prophylactic interventions are things that are done or medications that are given 'just in case', to prevent potential problems from occurring. Often, the situation or problem that they aim to prevent will only happen occasionally, but the intervention will be offered to many women or babies in the hope that the few who would have experienced the problem are among those who have taken up prophylactic treatment.

Prophylactic interventions do not themselves give information on the likelihood of a problem occurring, nor are they generally used with screening or other tests which could give information on this.

These interventions are often promoted as the medical equivalent of putting on a seatbelt before you get in a car or while the airplane is taxiing to the runway. Most people won't experience a crash or severe turbulence but, if you happen to be among the few people who do, you're protected. The key differences between seatbelts and medical forms of prophylaxis are that (a) the things they are seeking to protect you or your baby from can be very rare and (b) medical prophylaxis often has far greater potential to bring about side effects or to have other unwanted consequences than wearing a seatbelt does, so it's important that you are able to weigh up the pros and cons of each course of action for you.

The use of prophylactic interventions raises some bigger questions too. Is it appropriate to give these to all women or babies when only a few will benefit? Are there other ways of establishing whether a particular woman or baby is at risk? Are the side effects of prophylactic interventions justified for the women and babies who turn out not to have been at risk?

For instance, women used to be prevented from eating and drinking in labour because it was (wrongly) thought that this was dangerous for those who would end up having a caesarean section. But all of the women who were subject to this policy were then in danger of needing other intervention in their labour as they became hungry, thirsty, tired and in need of the greater reserves of energy that they would have had if they had been able to eat and drink.

In systems of maternity care, where policies are made in order to manage the movement of thousands of women through the system every year, prophylactic interventions are often promoted because there is seen to be an overall benefit on a population level. But you are an individual, not a population statistic so, again, it's up to you to decide whether or not these are right for you and your baby and family.

Examples of prophylactic interventions used in modern maternity care include vitamin K (for babies), anti-D for rhesus negative women, antibiotics (for a number of possible reasons including Group B Strep carriage or preterm labour), routine induction of labour, routine medical management of the birth of the placenta and routine cord care.

Questions to consider with prophylactic interventions

I use the acronym PIEDAY to help people remember the questions to ask of prophylactic interventions.

P for Problem.

What problem is this trying to prevent? What are the consequences of the problem? If I decline prophylaxis and I or my baby experience the problem, what (if anything) can be done to deal with it at that point?

I for Incidence.

What percentage of women or babies would end up with the problem if no-one had prophylaxis?

E for Effectiveness.

How well does the prophylactic intervention work? In how many cases does it do what it is designed to do?

D for Downsides.

What are the risks or side effects of the prophylactic intervention for me and/or my baby?

A for Alternatives.

Are there alternatives to the prophylaxis, e.g. herbs,

supplements, other things that we could try which might have a similar effect but with fewer downsides?

Y for 'what's right for You?'

Do some women and babies have a higher chance of experiencing this problem than others? If so, am I in a group that is more or less likely to experience the problem? And how does all of this fit with my (or our) personal situation, beliefs, culture and preferences?

Elective interventions

Elective interventions describe things which may or may not be intended to restore someone's health or assist directly with the progress of pregnancy, birth or the postpartum and neonatal period, but which are used on request.

They may be requested by women themselves, or they may be offered as an option or a preference rather than because they are medically beneficial. The most common elective interventions are pain relief (of all kinds, from massage to epidural or spinal anaesthesia), elective caesarean section and elective induction of labour.

The use of water for labour and birth is a good example of an elective intervention, though it is worth knowing that the same intervention can be used electively in one context and as a clinical intervention in another. For instance, I have used water pools as a clinical intervention in situations where a woman is labouring in hospital and having trouble relaxing. Sometimes, getting into warm water can improve the rhythm of a woman's labour surges. But many times, women use a pool simply because the feeling of getting into a pool or bath during labour can be immensely relaxing and they find that it helps them cope better.

One of the most significant questions in relation to an

elective intervention is whether the woman herself wants this intervention or whether it is being recommended by a health care provider. If the woman herself wants (or is OK with) the elective intervention, it is also important to ensure that she is aware of all of the pros and cons that may be associated with it. This category of interventions, as you've no doubt already gathered, not only includes some of the most recent, modern technological interventions such as epidural and caesarean section but also some of those (such as using warm water and massage to relieve pain) which women have been choosing themselves since time immemorial.

The question of whether some of these interventions, especially elective caesarean section, can be or should be or is an option for all women is complex and it depends on where you are in the world and on who is looking after you. If you think that you may want certain elective interventions during the birth of your baby, then you may need to plan your setting and care provider accordingly. This is the same no matter whether you're hoping to avail yourself of the more technological interventions, such as epidural (in which case you'll need to be in a hospital that offers that) or whether you're seeking to use water for labour.

In the latter case, you may wish to check not only whether the setting where you plan to birth has a pool available, but how likely you are to be able to get in it. In some institutions, such facilities are in high demand and some women are disappointed because someone else is using the room when they arrive. In others, the pool turns out to be mostly for show, and women may be told that it is not possible for them to use it. It is also worth asking about the risk criteria for the pool, as some women are told that they may not use the pool because they are deemed to have a risk factor. In this case, if using a pool is important to you, you may wish to consider another place of birth, negotiate with the hospital or hire a pool to use at home before you go in.

Questions to consider with elective interventions

The BRAINS acronym can also be useful here, with one extra addition which we will come to at the end.

What are the Benefits?

Do I feel the use of this intervention will be of benefit to me, my baby or my birth experience? Does my caregiver think this will be beneficial? Is there evidence for this?

What are the Risks?

Are there any potential downsides? How do I feel about these? As before, is there a danger of a cascade of intervention that might not otherwise be needed?

What are the Alternatives?

What other options are open to me? Are the risks and benefits of those options more or less acceptable to me?

What does my Intuition tell me?

What's your gut feeling? What does your body tell you?

What if I do Nothing?

You may wish to consider the different pathways that are open to you, and think about the possible consequences or endpoints of each path. Which feels more OK to you?

Smile, Scuse yourself or ask for a Second opinion?

These questions may or may not be appropriate or necessary when you are requesting an elective intervention, but there are a couple of other words beginning with 's' that are good to remember when you are considering elective interventions. One of these is to ask whether the use of this intervention is standard and the other is to ask whether you need to do anything special to be able to access it.

Following your gut, intuition or feelings

This chapter of the book is one of the most detailed, and we have looked in depth at some complex ideas. There are a few more ideas in the next chapter but I want to just pause and offer a reminder that we all have different preferences in how we think and make decisions. Some people like to analyse things, and others prefer to just go with their gut rather than to ask lots of questions. I also know people who love having a detailed masterplan or, in some cases, giving their partner the task of studying this information and asking the right questions when the time comes.

Some people do both at different times, or they vary their approach to decision making depending on the situation. I think it's really important that woman and families have access to this kind of thinking so that they have the ability to engage in conversations about what's being offered and why. But I also think it's really important to get to the point where you feel able to let go, trust your body and go with your gut feeling or instinct. Although I have already mentioned intuition, body knowledge and even having a 'spidey sense' several times, I want to say a tiny bit more about that, as it's not something that is valued highly in our culture.

When somebody suggests something to you, you'll often find that you get an instant reaction somewhere in your body.

That may be a positive reaction, such as a happy or relieved feeling, or it may be that your tummy flips or you feel a bit sick or you feel revulsion.

I want to tell you that it can be OK to trust that feeling.

I'm not saying you should always follow it but, if you listen to it, it can often lead to good insight about whether something feels right for you or your baby. I would never argue that intuition is infallible, but I do know that our bodies can sometimes tell us things before it is possible to know them in other ways.

9. More on birth intervention: intention, indication and individualisation

In this chapter, I'm going to continue discussing tools for making decisions about birth interventions. One of the questions that I encounter quite often from women and their partners goes something like this:

"I've been told that I need an intervention, but I'm not really clear on what it is and why they're suggesting it. Where do I start in asking about why this is recommended for me and in figuring out whether it's a path I want to go down?"

Some people find it easy to use the information and questions in the previous chapter to figure out what kind of intervention they are being offered. But some people find this harder to work out, so a slightly different approach involves a mnemonic that uses three 'I's; intention, indication and individualisation. If you make a note of these three words and use them to ask questions about what you're being offered, the answers should help you to figure out what kind of intervention is on offer. This in turn should, I hope, help guide you to the right questions to ask so you can make the decision that's right for you.

Intention (the 'what')

The first question to ask is what kind of intervention you're being offered. Sometimes that might be obvious, but it isn't always. Plus, as I said in chapter 7, some interventions can fall under different categories at different times. In the vast majority of cases the intervention you're being offered will fall into one of the first three categories that I described in chapter 7 (that is, screening tests, clinical interventions or prophylactic interventions), so ask something like:

"I'm trying to understand what we're being offered here. Is this a screening test, a form of prophylaxis, or are you suggesting that we need intervention because something isn't going to plan?"

You might think that the why (which we're coming to next) is the most important question, and it is definitely a crucial one. But the reason that I have written so much about the different types of intervention and the reason I have put the 'what' first is that having an understanding of what kind of intervention you're looking at can tell you exactly what questions you need to consider, and I know from long experience that this can really help.

Do bear in mind, though, that not all practitioners will be aware of this way of thinking, and they might not be immediately able to tell you which category an intervention falls into. I know that might be surprising but, while some practitioners think very deeply about what they're doing and why, others don't, or else they may have been educated to focus on getting tasks done rather than thinking about why they needed to do them. If the professional doesn't immediately know, that's not necessarily a huge problem. You've got all the information you need, in chapter 7, to be able to figure this out and if you ask a few basic questions about what the thinking behind offering a particular intervention is; you'll be able to work out for yourself which follow-on questions to ask or to look up.

Indication (the 'why')

In medical terms, the word indication refers to the reason(s) for recommending a test, procedure, drug or intervention. When doctors perform an operative procedure such as caesarean section, they will record the indication; for instance caesarean section for fetal distress, or caesarean section at maternal request.

Asking what the indication for a particular test or recommendation is can be helpful in enabling you to understand what someone sees as the key issue or problem.

That should give you a good starting point from which to ask other questions, and it can often be very helpful to know why the practitioner thinks that something will help give information or be beneficial for you or your baby. They've got more experience of using such tests and interventions, but their beliefs or ethical standpoint might differ from yours, so the more you can find out about their basis for offering the intervention, the better placed you are to start thinking about whether it's right for you and your family.

You are looking for a clear, specific and (as we'll discuss more in a moment) individualised reason for something being recommended as useful. Be aware that sometimes you will not be given a clear indication, or you may be told that there are several factors in the equation. I can tell you from my experience that some situations truly are complex and intervention is offered or suggested because there are two or three different causes of concern without their being one key problem that someone can put their finger on. But if the answer you receive is defensive, muddled, patronising or you feel that someone is trying to scare you (and your gut feeling or intuition will often tell you this), then you might want to step back from the situation, take some time to discuss your options with your family and/or ask for another opinion.

Individualisation (the 'who')

It can also be helpful to find out whether you're being offered an intervention because your care provider thinks there is a specific and individualised reason to offer it in your unique personal circumstances, or whether the intervention is offered to all women or babies at a certain time or under a certain set of circumstances. In other words, is this a routine intervention, which might warrant a bit more thinking about (because it may or may not be useful in your specific circumstances), or is the suggestion that intervention might be warranted already specifically tailored to your situation? There can be a huge difference. Some women, of course, are very happy to have the standard package of care that is offered to everyone, but others aren't.

Do be aware that some tests and interventions are offered to certain groups of women or babies, for instance small babies, women who have a particular blood type, older women, larger-than-average women or women who have had fertility treatment. This doesn't mean that they are being offered on an individual basis. It means that they are being offered to everyone who falls into a particular group or category. When systems of care are trying to help thousands of women to have babies every year, it is understandable that they need to develop policies based on what might be good across the whole population, but that still doesn't necessarily mean that their suggestion will point to the path that is right for you. On the other hand, it might be the perfect path for you, but it doesn't hurt to ask a few questions so you can be sure of that before you agree.

10. Real-life birth decision making

Let's put the theory aside and look at a few examples of real life decision making. The first three examples are all on the same topic, the decision about whether or not to have vitamin K given to a newborn baby, and they are taken from my book (Wickham 2017). The contrast between them shows how different people have different priorities and how this affects people's decision making even when they all have the same information. After that, I have tried to pick some varied stories to illustrate different elements of decision making.

Cybele

Cybele and her partner decided not to give vitamin K to their baby Emily when they realised that vitamin K deficiency bleeding was very rare. Cybele said she also felt the same about testing for Group B strep bacteria. When she shared her story with me, she wrote that, *"In both cases, we're talking about something really rare and yes, I know it can be fatal and yes I know she could have been the one in twelve thousand, or even more rare with GBS, I think, but what would the consequences of giving vitamin K or taking antibiotics be? People say you'll do anything to protect your baby, and of course you will, but it's no good only thinking one dimensionally."*

For Cybele, the bigger picture was important. She wanted to think very widely about the decisions that she and her partner needed to make for her pregnancy and their baby and, as she says, it was important to her to think about the consequences of different courses of action.

Ella

When Ella describes the decision that she made about vitamin K, it's clear that she has a different take on the issues from Cybele. Ella's words suggest that she was happy to follow the population-level recommendation about vitamin K and other interventions and to put her trust in the people caring for her rather than to spend time questioning and looking through the evidence for herself. Ella wrote, *"I didn't want to take any chances so yes, we had the vitamin K. I don't see why you wouldn't, as they can die if you don't. We did most things they suggested. They are the experts, so they know best."*

Ella sits firmly and happily in the technocratic viewpoint, and has no great desire to challenge what is offered. Which is great: the really important thing here is that both Cybele and Ella made the decision that was right for their families.

Olivia

Olivia is a midwife who shared the story of a woman for whom she cared. A key message here is that sometimes there exist options that we might not initially be offered, perhaps because no-one has thought about them. But it's OK to think outside the box and to ask about other alternatives.

"As a midwife, I once cared for a lady who made a choice I had never thought about with regard to vitamin K prophylaxis for her baby. She had a child already, who had inadvertently been given a massive overdose of vitamin K (not in the UK), and experienced a stroke in the neonatal period which had left her with weakness on one side. No one was willing to say it was or wasn't because of the vitamin K. She had a PhD, so was very confident in analysing research papers and making decisions. Her choice was to have the vitamin K prophylaxis given to the baby intramuscularly at discharge from midwifery care, which because she had independent midwifery care was when the baby was a few weeks old (not at 10 days like in the NHS). Her rationale was that early onset VKDB was almost always associated with maternal conditions or medications; medium onset was usually mild, but late onset was the one to be slightly worried about. She went on to have another baby, this time within NHS maternity care, and made the same decision again."

Corinne and Anna

I met Corinne and Anna about twenty years ago, and at that time it was more unusual than it is now to find same-sex couples openly having a baby together. The couple had decided that Corinne would give birth to their first baby and they were initially planning a hospital birth, but became quite frustrated after a few antenatal appointments because they felt that they were spending more time explaining their own situation to health professionals than on the questions and concerns that were bothering them.

Corinne approached me to talk about whether and how independent midwifery care would be different from the care they were receiving in the system, and she and Anna soon realised that this kind of care was right for them. Unlike many couples who decide to have independent midwifery care, however, this had very little to do with any beliefs they had about home birth, and everything to do with a desire to be cared for by someone who knew them and who wasn't going to ask them lots of questions about their situation which they felt were too personal and not relevant to their care.

People whose circumstances might be considered unusual or who are in the public eye often seek independent midwifery care for similar reasons, but what I really want to illustrate with this example is how decisions about care providers aren't always based on issues such as place of birth, but often on social or personal issues that are really important to a couple or family.

Gemma

Gemma really wanted a home birth and had read extensively around the subject of birth. She met with the local midwife for some antenatal care, but ended up feeling that she wanted to give birth on her own. Unlike some women, however, who decide to have an unassisted birth because they feel they cannot get the care that they want from local caregivers, this was (and remains) a positive choice for Gemma. She feels that birth is not a medical event and that she was better off being at home with just her husband, as her labour wasn't measured or monitored and this allowed her to birth peacefully and in her own time.

If you'd like to read a longer story about a woman's decision to experience an undisturbed birth, Australian GP Sarah Buckley tells her story of giving birth to her fourth baby at home with just her family in her book, Gentle Birth, Gentle Mothering (Buckley 2009).

Claire

Claire experienced a relatively calm and uneventful pregnancy until she began to bleed during her second trimester. Investigations showed that her placenta was partially covering her cervix, which meant that she would be in danger of bleeding when her cervix started to stretch. Her obstetrician recommended keeping a very close eye on her, with the recommendation that, if Claire continued to bleed, she might be wise to stay in hospital until the baby was born by caesarean section.

The bleeding stopped for a good few weeks, which was a big relief for Claire, and she took time to seek out lots of information about her situation from doctors, midwives, books and the internet. Claire came to the conclusion that a caesarean section really was the only option, but she realised that there were things that she really wanted. Claire developed a birth plan for her caesarean and this was negotiated with the consultant midwife and the obstetricians at her local hospital so that her baby's birth would include the things that were important to Claire and her husband. These included the music that was played while the surgery was performed, limiting the number of people in the operating theatre, asking those present to speak in quiet voices, ensuring that the baby was put straight onto Claire's chest and having lots of time for skin-to-skin cuddling. Stories like

Claire's are important because they illustrate how, even if circumstances mean that plan B or plan C come into play, there are still ways that birth can be personalised so that it fits with the needs and wants of a woman and her family.

Bella and Jack

I met Bella and Jack in a childbirth education setting, and Jack became one of the biggest fans of the tools that I shared in chapters 8 and 9. He loved being able to help Bella by analysing the options that they were offered in pregnancy, and always asked great questions. When Bella and Jack returned to the group with their new baby and told the story of Bella's labour and birth, Jack was also excited to share how he had used the BRAINS tool.

Bella's labour had slowed a bit towards the end, perhaps because she was tired, and their birth centre midwife had offered a series of suggestions which involved getting up and walking around, having some juice and dancing with the aid of a rebozo shawl. Jack applied the BRAINS tool and explored the pros and cons these ideas with the midwife and with Bella, but he soon realised, mainly through reading signs learned during his long relationship with Bella, that she really just wanted some rest. He negotiated this with the midwife, and Bella got back into the birth pool, in a position in which she could doze on Jack's shoulder when she was able to, and they agreed that they would dim the lights and just give Bella rest for an hour before doing anything else.

One of the things that Jack was really struck by was that, even though the birth centre midwife had presented options that were an alternative to the pharmacological augmentation that they would likely have been offered on the labour ward, resting was an alternative to the alternative. This, said Jack, was absolutely the best decision for them because about forty minutes after she settled down to rest, Bella asked for a cup of tea, drank one mouthful, brought it back up and then gave birth so quickly that the rest of the tea was still warm enough to drink while she was cuddling their newborn son.

This story is also a great illustration of how listening to a woman's body is so beneficial, whether that listening comes from the woman herself or via an insightful and attentive partner who knows their lover so well that they can help them to get what they need in labour.

Jenna and Dev

Quite a few years ago, I wrote about the experience of a past midwifery client, Jenna, who allowed me to share elements of her care story in a book chapter (Wickham 2006). Jenna and her partner Dev (who, for reasons that Jenna and I never quite got to the bottom of, insisted on picking a pseudonym which celebrated the owner of the corner shop in a certain British soap opera) had been through a journey of decision-making around so-called post-term pregnancy. They had decided to have a home birth and wanted to avoid intervention unless it was really the only safe option. Years later, I unexpectedly reconnected with Jenna and she reflected on her story in a way that allowed me to discuss elements of it even more deeply, so I will end this section with the longer story of Jenna's experience, which will allow us to explore further elements of real-life decision making.

Jenna needed to make a decision about whether or not she accepted the offer of routine induction of labour because her pregnancy had gone on for longer than average. The local guideline was to recommend that women had their labours induced once they were a certain number of days past their 'due date'. Jenna wasn't keen on this course of action and wanted to explore it further. I was well aware that this was one of the many areas of maternity care where the evidence didn't really show much of a benefit to intervention and in which the norm is not necessarily the best for everyone, or what everyone wants. (For the sake of full disclosure, I went on to look at this area for my PhD, and I've written several articles and books about it, including one to help women make decisions about induction of labour (Wickham 2018) but Jenna's pregnancy occurred before that time).

Together, Jenna, Dev and I worked through the various questions that they had, and I encouraged them to look for information and evidence from other sources as well. At the time, I described our interaction as 'a spiralling series of conversations' and I think that's a useful thing to know, because such decisions don't always get made on the spot, or in one conversation. Often, we need time to think, and sometimes to gather information from other sources.

Jenna and Dev became interested in the fact that many women have their labours induced because of a cultural belief that it is important that babies do not wait too long after their due date when, in fact, there is barely any difference between the outcomes for babies born to healthy women whose labour is induced and those for babies whose mothers decide to wait. They knew from friends that some of those same women reveal afterwards that they intuitively felt their baby wanted to stay inside a little longer. They had heard some negative experiences about women who had decided to have induction, but of course they didn't want to take any chances with their baby, so they were reassured to read the evidence and see that induction wasn't as beneficial as many people think it is. So it's possible to see how their pre-existing beliefs shaped their decision making, but they also discovered new information along the way.

There are a couple of aspects of Jenna and Dev's story which I think are particularly useful to share here, because they further illustrate the reality of making these decisions. First, it was in writing about Jenna and Dev's story that I first started paying attention to the importance of being really clear about what is being decided when decisions are made. Because even the women and families who decline interventions are not necessarily wanting to decline the intervention completely or to say that they would never have it under any circumstances. Instead, they are saying that they do not want to have it routinely, or in the absence of an individualised, good reason for them to have it. And, although it shouldn't be necessary to spell that out to health care professionals, I feel it's only fair to say that, sometimes, it can be helpful to do so.

Jenna decided to continue her pregnancy and decline routine induction of her labour; an approach that midwives often describe as 'watchful waiting'. We were paying careful attention and watching for any sign of an issue. But even when they declined routine induction, Jenna and Dev remained open to considering it if an issue arose. This isn't an uncommon stance to take. Many of the parents who decline routine vitamin K would be more than happy to have it if their baby had a problem which indicated that they might be at higher risk. I have also cared for several women who had decided to have a physiological placental birth rather than an actively managed third stage but who were more than happy to have drugs to facilitate the birth of the placenta and stop bleeding when they lost more blood than average.

The point is that it is not always about yes/no, accept/decline dichotomies. Often, there is a middle ground, where you don't have to decide between yes and no. As in the examples in chapters 8 and 9, you almost always also have the option of saying, *'actually, we'd like to wait an hour'* (or a week, or however long you would like to wait, as long as all is well) and revisit the decision again then. It is perfectly acceptable to make the decision that, rather than declining intervention outright, you are seeking a more individualised kind of care which includes deciding to have those very same interventions if needed rather than on a routine basis.

The second aspect of Jenna and Dev's story that I'd like to highlight is a realisation that Jenna had:

"I remember our journey side-tracking a lot, you know, like winding off onto other paths ... and some were interesting but not really helpful, and some were useful ... some were just dead-ends! And I do remember one evening, when it seemed like I was going round in circles and then Dev said something like, "you know, it seems like you just have to choose one route and then go with it,

because by not choosing you're actually choosing to wait, even if you're just waiting another few minutes while you think and talk some more, so if it's in your heart to wait then why not just choose that road for as long as it feels good and then you can relax and enjoy it?" That was the realisation point for me." (Wickham 2006)

Jenna gave birth to an eight-and-a-half-pound baby boy at daybreak when she was 43 weeks and (just) 2 days pregnant. Even now, as that baby is considering which university to go to, his mum still talks about the process of her decision making, and how much she learned about herself and about life from that experience. That's just one of the reasons that I make the claim, as I did in the beginning of the book, that the decisions that we make can shape our lives. Jenna and Dev's story wasn't straightforward. Jenna came under quite a lot of pressure from family and friends, especially when her pregnancy went past 42 weeks. At one point, they resorted to unplugging the phone in order to escape from the pressure. But Jenna says, even now, that the act of making that decision herself was one of the most important things she ever did. And that's not, she says, because she chose to decline intervention. It's because she made the decision herself, rather than having it made for her by a policy, or a guideline, or a healthcare provider. The strength and the sense of self-worth that this gave her, she says, is beyond measure.

References, resources and reading

This section of the book contains the references of all of the papers and books to which I have referred and suggestions of other books which offer information on elements of birth decision making or related topics. There's a bit of overlap between the two lists, because some books come under both of these headings.

Some of the books in the further reading list are a few years old, but I have included them because they are classics which contain information and a perspective not always offered by newer texts. I've tried to include a range of books and approaches and not everything will be to everyone's taste. Some are very academic and some are very chatty. Some are more evidence-based than others. They are suggestions and I recommend looking at the book blurb and some online reviews first to see what looks interesting and relevant to you.

A small number of appendices follow these lists. A few of these appendices are original and I have included them to give you a bit more information on some of the issues discussed in these pages. A few are adapted from blog posts relevant to the topics in this book. I have popped them in here to save you having to go online to find them but I do want to stress that these are only a handful of the posts that are available, and there are plenty more on my website, www.sarawickham.com, should you find yourself wanting more. The website has also a search box which you can use to find information on specific topics and, if you are a midwife, student, birth worker or someone wanting to enter that world, a free monthly newsletter which offers updates on the latest birth-related research and thinking.

References

Anonymous (2017). Informed consent in theatre. TPM 29(11): 47-50.

Beech BAL (2014). Am I Allowed? London: AIMS.

Berhan Y & Haileamlak A (2015). The risks of planned vaginal breech delivery versus planned Caesarean section for term breech birth: a meta-analysis including observational studies. British Journal of Obstetrics and Gynaecology DOI: 10.1111/1471-0528.13524

Birthplace in England Collaborative Group (2011). Perinatal and maternal outcomes by planned place of birth for healthy women with low risk pregnancies: the Birthplace in England national prospective cohort study. BMJ 343:d7400. doi.org/10.1136/bmj.d7400

Birthrights, 2013. Consenting to treatment. Available at: http://www.birthrights.org.uk/library/factsheets/Consenting-to-Treatment.pdf

Buckley S (2009). Gentle birth, gentle mothering. Celestial Arts.

Davis-Floyd RE (2004). Birth as an American Rite of Passage. University of California Press.

Davis-Floyd RE (2001). The Technocratic, Humanistic, and Holistic Paradigms of Childbirth. International Journal of Gynecology and Obstetrics 75(1): S5-S23.

MBRRACE-UK (2016) Perinatal Mortality Surveillance Report UK Perinatal Deaths for Births from January to December 2014 https://www.npeu.ox.ac.uk/downloads/files/mbrrace-uk/reports/MBRRACE-UK-PMS-Report-2014.pdf

Murphy-Lawless, Jo (1998). Reading Birth and Death: A history of obstetric thinking. Cork, Cork University Press.

NICE (2014). Intrapartum Care. National Institute for Clinical Excellence. https://www.nice.org.uk/guidance/cg190/chapter/1-recommendations

Prusova K, Tyler A, Churcher L and Lokugamage AU (2014). Royal College of Obstetricians and Gynaecologists guidelines: How evidence-based are they? 1-6. Journal of Obstetrics and Gynaecology 34(8): 706–711. doi:10.3109/01443615.2014.920794

Royal College of Obstetricians and Gynaecologists (2013). Induction of labour at term in older mothers. RCOG. www.rcog.org.uk/global assets/documents/guidelines/scientific-impact-papers/sip_34.pdf

Sartwelle TP and Johnston JC (2015). 'Cerebral palsy litigation: change course or abandon ship'. J Child Neurology 30(7): 828-41.

Sartwelle TP and Johnston JC (2016). 'Neonatal encephalopathy 2015: opportunity lost and words unspoken'. The Journal of Maternal-Fetal and Neonatal Medicine, 29(9): 1372-1375.

Schwartz C, Groww MM, Heusser P et al (2016). Women's perceptions of induction of labour outcomes: results of an online survey in Germany. Midwifery 35: 3-10.

UNICEF (2018). Research on skin-to-skin contact.
https://www.unicef.org.uk/babyfriendly/news-and-research/baby-friendly-research/research-supporting-breastfeeding/skin-to-skin-contact/

WHO (2018). Optimal timing of cord clamping for the prevention of iron deficiency anaemia in infants. http://www.who.int/elena/titles/cord_clamping/en/

Wagner M (2000). Technology in birth: first do no harm.
https://www.midwiferytoday.com/articles/technologyinbirth.asp

Wickham S (2006). Jenna's care story: post-term pregnancy. In Page LA & McCandlish R (2006). The New Midwifery: Science and Sensitivity in Practice. (second edition). Churchill Livingstone.

Wickham S (2009). Post-term pregnancy: the problem of the boundaries. MIDIRS Midwifery Digest 19(3): 463-69.

Wickham S (2010). Journeying with women: holistic midwives and relationship. Birthspirit Midwifery Journal (6):15-21.

Wickham S (2018). Inducing Labour: making informed decisions. (second edition). Birthmoon Creations.

Wickham S (2019). Group B Strep Explained. (second edition). Birthmoon Creations.

Further reading

Arms S (1994). Immaculate Deception II: myth, magic and birth. Celestial Arts.

Balaskas J (1992). Active Birth: The New Approach to Giving Birth Naturally. Harvard Common Press.

Banks M (1998). Breech Birth Woman Wise. BirthSpirit Ltd.

Beech BAL (2014). Am I Allowed? London: AIMS.

Buckley S (2009). Gentle birth, gentle mothering. Celestial Arts.

Davis E and Pascali-Bonaro D (2010). Orgasmic Birth: your guide to a safe, satisfying and pleasurable birth experience. Rodale Press.

Davis-Floyd RE (2017). Ways of Knowing About Birth: Mothers, Midwives, Medicine, & Birth Activism. Waveland Press.

Edwards NP (2005). Birthing Autonomy: women's experiences of planning home births. Routledge.

England P and Horowitz R (1998). Birthing from within: An Extra-Ordinary Guide to Childbirth Preparation. Partera Press.

Fletcher S (2014). Mindful Hypnobirthing: Hypnosis and Mindfulness Techniques for a Calm and Confident Birth. Vermilion.

Gaskin IM (2002). Spiritual Midwifery. The Farm Publishing Co.

Gaskin IM (2008). Ina May's Guide to Childbirth. Vermilion.

Goer K and Romano A (2013). Optimal care in childbirth: the case for a physiologic approach. Pinter & Martin.

Graves K (2017). The Hypnobirthing Book. Katharine Publishing.

Hill M (2017). The Positive Birth Book: A New Approach to Pregnancy, Birth and the Early Weeks. Pinter and Martin.

Hill M (2014). Water Birth: Stories to inspire and inform. Lonely Scribe.

Howell M (2009). Effective Birth Preparation: Your Practical Guide to a Better Birth. Intuition UN.

Kitzinger S (2012). Birth and sex: the power and the passion. Pinter and Martin.

Klaus MH, Kennell JH, and Klaus PH (2012). The Doula Book: how a trained labor companion can help you have a shorter, easier, and healthier birth. Da Capo Lifelong Books.

Lokugamage A (2011). The heart in the womb. Docamali.

Mongan M (2016). Hypnobirthing: The Mongan Method. Souvenir Press.

Murphy-Lawless, Jo (1998). Reading Birth and Death: A history of obstetric thinking. Cork, Cork University Press.

Odent M (1994). Birth Reborn: what birth should be. Souvenir Press.

Odent M (2007). Birth and Breastfeeding: Rediscovering the Needs of Women During Pregnancy and Childbirth. Clairview Books.

Osterholzer K (2018). A midwife in Amish country. Dreamscape Media.

Reed, B (2016). Birth in Focus. Pinter and Martin.

Simkin P (2017). The Birth Partner, 4th Edition, completely revised and updated: A complete guide to childbirth for dads, doulas, and other labor companions. Harvard Common Press.

Wickham S (2017). Vitamin K and the Newborn. Birthmoon Creations.

Wickham S (2018). Inducing Labour: making informed decisions. (second edition). Birthmoon Creations.

Wickham S (2019). Group B Strep Explained. (second edition). Birthmoon Creations.

Appendix 1: How to get more information about your birth rights

I am aware that this book will be read by people in many different countries and that the structure of health services varies widely around the world. The amount of choice that people have also varies widely, not just because of regional geographical, political or economic differences, but as a result of income, education, ethnicity and other factors. This is absolutely not OK and I would encourage anybody who cares about the wellbeing of women, babies and families to read lots and get involved in creating awareness and change.

In an ideal world, every care provider would ensure that all women were fully informed about all of their options, their rights and the possible pathways that they could take. Indeed, many women and families won't need or want to look further than their care provider for relevant information, which is great. So your care provider is a good first 'port of call', but some people will not yet have a care provider or may not feel that they have enough information from their care provider and will want to look further afield. Some women may have care providers who would like to help more but do not have the time, freedom or ability to do so.

These days, the internet is one of the best sources of information about women's birth rights on a local or national level. There are many groups, organisations and lists set up to share information online. In this appendix, I have included information for organisations that I know about and whose principles I know to be woman-centred. I would be happy to expand this list to include other organisations if anyone would like to send suggestions for inclusion in later editions of this book.

There are a few organisations which are specifically focused on women's birth rights. The best source of information about birth rights in the UK, for instance, is the organisation Birthrights (who can be found online at http://www.birthrights.org.uk/). They produce and update a whole series of factsheets on different topics which are available online. Another useful UK-based organisation is the Association for Improvement in the Maternity Services. AIMS' website is www.aims.org.uk and, in Ireland, AIMS Ireland offer resources, news and campaigning at http://aimsireland.ie/

In the US, Childbirth Connection offer information and factsheets at www.childbirthconnection.org/, including a useful leaflet entitled 'The Rights of Childbearing Women' which can be found at www.nationalpartnership.org/ research-library/maternal-health/the-rights-of-childbearing -women.pdf

Often, pregnancy, birth, parenting or infant feeding related organisations run by women, birth workers (such as doulas, childbirth educators and breastfeeding supporters) and/or health professionals such as midwives and doctors can offer information, even if their primary focus doesn't quite match what you're looking for. A good example of what I mean by this is homebirth organisations such as Homebirth Australia (http://homebirthaustralia.org/) and Homebirth Aotearoa (https://homebirth.org.nz/). These kinds of organisations tend to be run by people who are very knowledgeable about women's rights and what is available within their country or area, even if you are not looking to birth at home.

If you are looking online for information, it can sometimes help to search for similar key words and phrases, for example, 'human rights', 'women's rights', 'reproductive rights' and 'childbirth rights'. Do search – both online and on local community noticeboards or gathering places - for local or national homebirth groups, doulas, childbirth educators, information on hypnobirthing, pregnancy yoga teachers and anything else pregnancy-related that you can think of. People who are interested in birth and related issues are often good at networking and sometimes you just need to find one starting point and then you'll have a way into lots of information. Don't forget parenting, postnatal and/or breastfeeding groups or supporters, postnatal yoga teachers and baby massage or similar groups. These are the people who have just been on the journey (or who support the people who have just been on the journey) and they can also be a good source of knowledge.

In some countries, home educators' groups, alternative community organisations or healthy living organisations can be a good source of support or information. Midwifery-focused organisations may also be a source of information, but this can vary a bit. Many countries have midwifery colleges or official organisations, but some of these tend to be focused on organising or regulating midwives. But there are a number of companies (like the US-based Midwifery Today magazine at www.midwiferytoday.com) and organisations (such as the UK-based Association of Radical Midwives at www.midwifery.org.uk) who will have websites and social media pages which you might find useful.

Appendix 2: How to change your care provider

At several points throughout this book, I have pointed out that one possible course of action, if there is a mismatch between your views and desires and those of your care provider, is to seek a different care provider. I am well aware that this is easier for some people than others, for all the reasons that I've already mentioned in appendix 1; different systems of health care, different levels of access and privilege and so on.

It isn't just as simple as saying that those who have access to private health care (whether or not that is the main option in their area) have more choice, however. In Australia and the USA, for example, some women find it difficult to access the care that they want or to make the decisions that are right for them even through private means, because of constraints placed upon midwives' practice. In New Zealand, however, women are afforded a higher level of autonomy by the laws and regulations governing health care practice and are given information about their rights and about how to change care provider if they wish to do this.

In Canada, the USA and Australia, amongst other countries, choice is further limited by the fact that there are many more midwives in some areas than others. All over, women and families who live in remote and rural areas may find that they have fewer options although, somewhat ironically, some women living in rural areas report that they are sometimes more able to make the decisions that are right for them than their friends who live in cities.

In the UK, women who seek care within the National Health Service are allocated a midwife (although this is not to imply that they see the same midwife every time, because frequently women report rarely seeing the same midwife twice) and most have no idea whether it is even possible to ask for someone else. There exists what is known as a 'postcode lottery', where the kind of care that women receive differs vastly between different regions, and recent restrictions placed upon UK independent midwives mean that it is no longer possible to access independent midwifery care in the way that it used to be.

It can be seen from the way I have laid out these differences that it can be important to begin by gaining an understanding of how care is organised in your area. For that, I would refer you back to appendix 1, which should help you to find resources and information specific to your part of the world. But I also have a few general suggestions which I hope will help anyone who feels that they haven't yet found the care provider who is right for them.

1. **If you are in an area where you can choose, do some research and find out what your options are.** Look in local directories and online to see who is offering care locally. Ask people about their experiences. Read reviews (while bearing in mind that people are sometimes more likely to write about poor experiences than amazing ones). Take opportunities to go to events where you can meet care providers informally. Make an appointment with the care provider you feel drawn to and take along your questions.

2. **Even if you feel limited by cost or the nature of your health insurance, it's still worth finding out what the other options are.** Some women find that a care provider who is right for them doesn't cost as much as they thought. Some negotiate payment plans. Some have negotiated with insurance companies (or found loopholes) and some have decided the extra cost is worth it. I acknowledge that, for some, no cost is affordable, however.

3. **If you have chosen or been allocated a care provider who you do not feel is right for you, consider talking to them about it.** You can explain that, while you have nothing against them as a person, you feel that you would prefer to have a different care provider. I know that some people are worried about doing this, but a reasonable professional should be able to cope with it and understand that your comfort is the most important thing.

4. **If you are in an area (such as the UK) where you are allocated a care provider within a system of care, you still have options.** Talk to your care provider and ask whether other options or patterns of care are available. If you want to change your care provider for antenatal (pregnancy) care, then changing your GP is one option. If there is somewhere else that you would rather go for care during labour and birth (such as another hospital, maternity unit or birth centre or a team of midwives who offer continuity of care), you might want to approach them to ask about the options for transferring care. Some Trusts employ one or more consultant midwives, who can be very helpful in such situations. Check the hospital website or call the switchboard and ask if there is a consultant midwife to whom you can speak. You can also write or speak to the head of midwifery or a midwifery manager. Other options for support include local groups, for example a Maternity Voices Partnership (in England), a Maternity Services Liaison Committee (MSLC) in Scotland, Wales or Northern Ireland or a Patient Advice and Liaison Service (often shortened to PALS). If speaking to people in person or on the phone doesn't make a difference, try writing. Seek information, support and advice from local groups or organisations or from birth activists, as in appendix 1.

5. **If your concerns or wishes are rooted in a religious, spiritual or philosophical preference or belief, be open and honest about that.** In many countries, cultural safety is considered to be very important and your wishes should be respected. I am often surprised at how much easier it is for women and families to negotiate a change if their wish is based in a religious belief than if they state it as a preference.

6. **Remember: you deserve care that is appropriate, respectful and right for you.** It can feel awkward to have a conversation with someone (although you don't always have to do that), but the really important thing is that you feel comfortable with the decisions that you are making, and that includes the person or people who will be caring for you.

Appendix 3: When consent is not consent

This appendix is a reworking of a blog post which is available on my website. I have included it here because it builds upon some of the issues discussed in chapter 3.

When is consent not consent?

That's not intended to be a trick question, though I'll admit it is a bit of a leading one because, although there are several possible answers to this, which are all more than worthy of debate, I am really only wanting to write about one today: the so-called consent that is sought when a midwife or doctor is halfway through a vaginal examination which a woman has agreed to and, out of the blue and before removing their fingers, asks the woman if she would like to have another procedure performed at the same time. The additional procedure is usually either the breaking of the baby's waters (which is also called ARM or artificial rupture of the membranes) or, in countries where intervention in pregnancy is greater than average and vaginal examination is carried out during pregnancy, a stretch and sweep. That's a procedure which forms part of induction of labour. As such, it needs to be properly discussed so that a woman can decide whether or not it is something she wants to have or not.

I was horrified to receive several emails from women who had experienced this happening. And, try as I might, I can't see how this kind of action is justifiable. It bothers me on so many levels, and I can't find a single angle to look at it from which doesn't lead to my concluding that it flies in the face of the notion of informed decision-making.

First, both of the procedures given as examples above (that is, ARM and stretch and sweep) might sound innocuous, but they are means of attempting to induce and/or augment (or speed up) labour. Some women might well decide they want to have them, after they have had a chance to think about them and weigh up the risks and benefits. But they are interventions, and women thus deserve to have that time to think about them, seek more information, consider their options and discuss them with loved ones.

None of which is possible or practical while one is in the middle of being intimately examined. In fact, the kind of thinking and deliberating required to make a decision might not even be possible or practical for some women while they are in the company of a waiting professional, though I acknowledge that this depends a lot on the relationship between the woman and attendant and that there are times when this might be unavoidable.

Generally, neither ARM or stretching and sweeping are emergency procedures, so speedy decision-making is not necessary. And many – perhaps most – women find vaginal examinations uncomfortable, embarrassing and/or painful. For some women, they are psychologically traumatic. Women will not always tell their attendants if that is the case, though. In some cases this might be because they do not know the attendant well enough to trust them, while for others this is because the only possible response for them is dissociation, which is where someone needs to focus their mind on something else in order to cope with a traumatic experience. Either way, they want the examination to be over as soon as possible. In some cases, a woman might agree to anything in order to get the examination to stop.

That is not informed decision-making.

I don't think that practitioners who do this are necessarily setting out to coerce or harm women. I can see how, from their perspective, they might genuinely think that it's kinder to save women from having an additional examination, or they might not have thought about the ramifications of this. That's partly why I wrote a blog post about this, to say to birth professionals: please, if you have ever done this, think about what it does to the women you care for. And don't do it again.

I am concerned from the emails I receive – which are not, by the way, limited to particular countries or types of professionals – that this is something which needs to be said. I cannot see how this is ever an appropriate time during which to discuss whether or not a woman wants to have an intervention which may have significant implications for her and her baby's experience, and I certainly do not think that it is a kind or ethical context in which to ask someone to make a decision.

If this happens to you, you are completely within your rights to tell the attendant to stop examining you before discussing any further decisions. Remember that it is your absolute right to say no or stop at any time.

Actually, that might be the most important sentence in this book, so I'm going to say it again and make it stand out.

Remember that it is your absolute right to say no or stop at any time.

A midwife friend of mine also recommends to women that they are very clear with the attendant before they consent to a vaginal examination that they are not consenting to any related intervention and that they do not want to discuss further interventions during the examination. I don't feel it is right that any woman should feel she has to be proactive in this way. I would much rather live in a world where all women could relax and trust everybody they met. But if you have any concerns about this, please know that you can be clear ahead of time and that you always have the right to say no or stop or to walk away.

Appendix 4: How to respond to fear-based information

One consequence of living in a technocratic world is that some people feel very fearful when people want to make decisions that are considered unusual or a bit alternative from the norm. As a midwife, I have a tendency to want to protect pregnant women from the harsher elements of this truth, but as an educator I know it's important that people are prepared for the possibility that they may encounter such attitudes.

So it is possible that you may encounter fear-based attitudes, and even what some people call 'shroud waving' or 'playing the dead baby card'. Both of these are horrible terms, and I apologise for using them, but they accurately describe what some women/couples face when they are told that, if they make a particular decision, their baby could die.

Often, this is not true, and it is a horrible way of trying to persuade people to comply with a recommended intervention like induction of labour or caesarean section. The only way that I know to help people deal with this is to ensure that women and their families are aware of the possibility that this might happen ahead of time, and to ensure that they feel strong and confident enough to respond to it.

How can you respond to such statements? Well one dad-to-be replied to the consultant who suggested that declining induction might lead to stillbirth by smiling and raising his eyebrows. *"Is that really true?"* he asked. *"Because someone told us you might say that, and I'd like the evidence please!"* In this situation, he used his strength of character to bounce the metaphorical ball right back to the doctor who used this threat, and it worked for him and his partner.

While travelling recently, I met a woman who also asked her doctor for evidence to support the allegation that her baby was five times more likely to die if she didn't do what he suggested. A week after she made her request, she and her husband kept an appointment with the same doctor who began their consultation with a heartfelt apology. He had looked for evidence to support the statement he had made, which he had picked up by listening to what was said to women by senior staff, only to find that it didn't exist. There was, in fact, no real difference in outcomes between the two possible paths that the woman could take in this situation.

Often, women themselves don't feel able to challenge care providers when they are pregnant, and this is one reason why it can be helpful to take your partner, a friend or a doula to appointments, but do have a conversation beforehand about how you would like them to behave/respond if this kind of conversation should take place.

Not everyone feels brave when confronted with such statements. But please know that they are often untrue and that they play on our modern fears about risk. There is no way that we can all inoculate ourselves from every risk; life is risky and no-one can promise you that everything will be OK if you take any particular path. But professionals (or anybody else, come to that) should not use fear to try and get you to go down the path that they think you should take. I would encourage you to be aware of this possibility and to be aware of your rights and some possible responses.

Some colleagues and I now suggest to women that, if faced with a professional who seems to be using this kind of threat, they should look the professional in the eye and ask them to provide a written guarantee that, if they follow the suggested advice, their baby will be born alive and healthy. This works, because it's not possible to make any guarantee about anything, and it's the most effective way that I know of responding to such treatment. Always remember that you are not obliged to do anything that you do not want to do and you can always walk out of a situation that is distressing you.

Appendix 5: Why we need to develop awareness of busy-ness

I've heard a few stories over the years from people processing decisions they made during labour and pondering what they might have done differently. Often (although of course not always), people who are thinking deeply about such issues are focused on wanting to grow and learn in a positive way rather than to blame or regret, and I have noticed a couple of trends. The one I want to talk about here is something that I have heard a few times, in one form or another. *"I wish I had worried less about how busy the staff were"*.

Anyone who has spent any time in hospitals delivering maternity care will know that, at times, they can be really busy. Some are really busy some of the time and some are really busy all of the time. In the UK for instance, maternity staff face ongoing increases in the number of women that they are expected to care for, often alongside a decrease in staff numbers and resources. This is echoed in many different countries, although the detail of the political and economic underpinnings varies.

Maternity staff also face increases in the expectations that are placed upon them, from many different directions, and anyone who manages to carry out their work without looking permanently frazzled is, quite frankly, heroic. So these people deserve understanding, compassion, love and, yes, all the chocolate that they receive from grateful parents, ideally alongside some serious lobbying of those who are putting them under this intolerable pressure.

So I am not writing this lightly or without consideration of the working lives of midwives, doctors and birth workers. I'm not suggesting that anyone should ignore or develop immunity to the busy-ness of others. But let's turn to the perspective of those seeking care in busy units and go back to the reflections that I mentioned at the beginning of this piece. Because I have, as I said, met a good many women and families who wish, after the fact, that they had been less focused on the busyness of the staff or ward.

A typical story is that an intervention or option is offered which the woman or couple aren't really sure about. They'd like to know more, but they know that their midwife is tired and looking after two other families, so they don't want to bother her. Or, they want to ask to wait and see how things go, but they fear that this will make the midwife's day harder, so they go along with what they think the midwife or doctor wants. Later, they wish they hadn't. Things didn't go the way they hoped, they feel that this was because they didn't make the decision that was right for them. This wish they hadn't been so nice or polite, or that they had been more assertive. Their learning is that, next time, they will focus more on their needs and not feel they have to comply because others are under pressure.

The message here is fairly simple: it's OK to ask for more time to discuss things; it's OK to ask for more information and it is your right to have all of these things. In fact, it's often advantageous and desirable to take a bit more time. (Staff will let you know if the situation really is time-critical). I could tell you lots of stories of situations where the 'stitch in time' proverb was true; where a bit more information or a five minute time-out to consider things might have saved a lot of hassle in the long run. But that would detract, I think, from the simple point I want to make here.

It's OK to ask for time and information, and it's also possible to do that in a respectful and compassionate way that honours the fact that staff may be busy. It's your birth, and your journey.

Appendix 6: How to cancel a labour induction

This appendix was also originally a blog post and I have included it in the book because it is one of the most recommended posts on my website. It was written for women in a UK context, but a lot of it will be relevant for women in other countries as well. If you'd like to know more about induction of labour, I have a whole book on this topic (Wickham 2018), but this post deals with a common query which is summarised by this question:

"I had an appointment with a consultant last week and was given a date for induction, although I wasn't really asked whether I wanted it and it was all very fast. There's no medical reason for inducing me, it's just that I'll be 41 weeks pregnant on that date. When I got home and thought about it and read more, I decided I wanted to cancel it. But how do I do that?"

Induction of labour is one of the most commonly searched-for topics on my website and a good number of people arrive on my site after searching for variations on the question, 'How to cancel a labour induction?' And in my workshops and courses, midwives and birth folk often tell stories about women who have been given an unwanted induction date, sometimes even sent by letter and generated by a computer rather than a person. So, with the usual disclaimers that this isn't midwifery or medical advice and that women need to make decisions based on a careful assessment of their individual situation and needs and ideally after a discussion with a woman-centred caregiver who understands their situation and needs, I felt this needed a bit of discussion.

Induction isn't compulsory

The 'how do I cancel an induction?' question is a sad indictment on the maternity services in the areas in which women are asking this question. It underlines the way in which many women don't feel that they are at the centre of or in control of their maternity care. I am both immensely grateful to Beverley Beech for writing her book Am I Allowed and immensely sad that she needed to write it. But in her words,

"Since most women simply assume they should, or feel obliged to, do as they are told – in their first pregnancy anyway – doctors and midwives, who are often busy, and who rarely encounter women who decline tests and interventions, assume that consent has been given. They are supposed to be offering and providing care, not insisting on it. The reason they want you to have a particular test or procedure may not be because of your individual need, but because it fits in with the hospital protocol. This is a set of written guidelines, which women rarely see, aimed at providing safe care for the majority, for that unit, and often not based on research. One size fits all, but it might not fit you. If in doubt, ask to see the protocol which applies to your type of care. You have a right to see it. And a right not to follow it." (Beech 2015: 1-2)

There are pros and cons of induction

Women and babies are individual and, because one size doesn't fit all, many midwives and birth folk feel frustrated that there exist recommendations about what all women should do, for instance at a particular stage of gestation. For a few women and babies, induction of labour is a life-saving intervention, and I absolutely understand that there are quite a few women who can't wait to have their babies and who are delighted at the idea of having their labour induced. But there are also women who would much rather go into labour on their own and who find the idea of excess intervention and being separated from their partners for the time it takes labour to get going (which can sometimes take a couple of days) not what they want. We know from research that most women who experience induction would not choose to be induced again in a future pregnancy (Schwartz et al 2016).

These days, induction is often recommended simply because a woman has reached a certain point in her pregnancy or because she or her baby are perceived to have a certain risk factor. But there often isn't good evidence to show that induction makes a significant difference to outcomes and, even if there was a difference, this is still the woman's decision to make. So why are systems still making population-level recommendations about the care of women and babies?

The first piece of advice that I offer to any woman (or family member) who is given an induction date that she isn't sure about is to ask questions and find out why induction is being recommended in their particular case. Is this a routine recommendation, or are there specific reasons why it is recommended for their particular situation at this stage of their pregnancy?

If you are told that induction is deemed to be a safer or better option than waiting for spontaneous labour in your case, you may wish to ask for an explanation of why this is, and/or to see the research on which this statement is based. Having said that, however, it is worth knowing that there IS research which concludes that induction is safer/better, but it isn't necessarily all good research. If you'd like to find out more about that, pop the word 'induction' into the search box on my website, and it will give you lots more resources to read.

Women/families are also entitled to ask for a second opinion. As above, there are sometimes really good reasons for recommending induction, but sometimes there are not. One size still doesn't fit all.

Were you involved in the discussion?

I am, sadly, hearing from some women who are given an appointment for induction without even having had a discussion about it, and from others who (in their words) felt that they were 'just told' that this was what was going to happen. In some areas of health care, there is a tendency for systems to automatically send or give out medical appointments that people may or may not want and have not been asked about, and I am also thinking here of friends and colleagues who have been mailed unwanted appointments for mammograms, cervical smear tests or other kinds of screening. Recently, I have heard this happening with induction of labour as well.

There are a number of reasons why, if you are managing a bureaucratic system, it is considered easier, better or more efficient to automate such things, but no amount of population-level justification will make it feel better to a person who is sad or upset that they are not being treated as the individual that they are.

I have also been really saddened to hear from more and more birth folk that women in their areas are now given an induction date almost as soon as their due date is calculated. In other cases, the due date and the induction date are automatically calculated by the ultrasound machinery, even if conception is known to have occurred on a different day (for instance because the baby was conceived through IVF or because the woman's husband is in the military and they only spent one night together in two months).

What on earth does this say to the women about our trust in their body's ability to grow, birth and feed their baby?

There are more than two options

It can be helpful to remind ourselves that most women pay for the health care that they receive, either directly, via insurance payments, via the work they do or through their or their family's tax payments. I'm not really a fan of thinking of ourselves as consumers, because it's not an appropriate comparison, but, when we access health care, we are the recipient of a service. I wish more women knew that care should be tailored to their needs, and that it doesn't have to be an all-or-nothing, stark black or white decision, as discussed in Jenna and Dev's story in chapter 10.

Many of the women who I've met who have questioned a recommendation of induction don't necessarily want to decline the induction outright and forever. They might instead want a different date, or to wait and see for another week. Or to be treated as an individual and negotiate the induction date that is right for them, not the one generated by the computer, which didn't take into account that they KNOW they conceived two weeks later than the date of their last menstrual period suggests.

Sometimes women want to discuss the decision with their partner or family rather than agreeing to a date straight away, or to gather information which will help them to know how the baby is doing before making a decision. None of this is unreasonable. As I have written elsewhere:

"It is quite reasonable for a woman to say, 'No, I do not want my labour induced at 41 weeks, but I would like an appointment at (say) 41 weeks and 5 days in order to talk about whether I may want to be induced at 42 weeks' or, 'I do not want my labour induced at this point but I will let my midwife know if I change my mind'" (Wickham 2014).

Again, it's an individual and personal decision.

The nuts and bolts of cancelling induction

So what to do to cancel the induction? Well, if women have a good relationship with a midwife or other caregiver, then the best way forward is for them to contact that midwife and share the decision with them. The midwife may have individualised information or suggestions to share, and will likely ensure that the woman has a timely antenatal appointment and ask her to get in touch if anything happens or if she changes her mind.

Not everyone has a midwife, though, and some of the stories I've been hearing are from women who either don't have a midwife (for instance, they're in a country where maternity care is obstetrician-led) or who have never seen the same midwife twice and don't feel that they have a good relationship with anyone. It's these women who are probably amongst those who search the internet on this question, as some of them just don't know who or where to call. What do they do? I know that some women decide to just ignore the induction date and not call anyone, but others are concerned that such action may have unwanted repercussions.

It also depends on what the woman feels she can deal with at that stage of pregnancy. I know of women who have taken control, called the hospital and politely and firmly explained that they do not need the appointment, and I know of women who have asked their partner or a friend to make the call instead, generally in the hope of keeping their stress levels down and their oxytocin levels up. Some women decide to text their midwife or doctor instead of calling, and others have phoned the antenatal clinic out-of-hours and left a message on the answerphone rather than calling a 24-hour service such as the labour ward where they would be talking directly to a member of staff. Some have heard nothing after leaving such a message and have simply turned up at the hospital a day or two later in spontaneous labour. No-one mentioned the induction date then or later. Other women who took that path have received a phone call from a staff member who questioned their decision and this, again, is why I am delighted that we have books such as Am I Allowed (Beech 2014) as well as organisations which help women know what their rights are and where to go if they need support.

In an ideal world, there would be no reason for this appendix. A woman would only be given an induction date if it was something she asked for or agreed to after discussion and she would know how change or cancel it. I have a dream that these women's phone calls would be answered by their friendly caseloading midwife who would ask how they were doing, how the baby was and chat through their decision in a friendly, relaxed way, ensuring the woman had up-to-date, individualised information. The midwife would have plenty of time to chat things through with the woman and her family, to make sure that the woman was OK and had all her questions answered and that they both had their next antenatal appointment on their calendars.

I hope one day I can delete this appendix because women only get given an induction date if it's something that they actively ask for after an individualised discussion of their needs.

Appendix 7: Three things I wish every woman knew about pregnancy and birth knowledge

This final appendix is another adapted blog post and some of what I have said in here (especially in the second point) can be found elsewhere in this book. But not all, and there are some positive thoughts in here that I would like to share, so here's a bonus piece which summarises some of the already-discussed issues and adds a few other thoughts into the mix.

Ask any midwife, doctor or birth worker what three things they wish they could tell all women, and you'll probably get three statements that tell you as much about the writer's passion and beliefs as about birth. My list is no exception. I could tell you I wished every woman knew that they didn't need to buy every baby product in sight, and I do wish that, but not nearly as much as I wish these three things, which reflect my passion for understanding different kinds of birthing knowledge and the ways they relate to each other.

1. During the last century or so, a number of developments in society and technology have undermined women's birthing knowledge.

I'm not suggesting that this is a long-term intentional plot whose intricate details are hidden in some secret code on banknotes and in the relative location of maternity hospitals to ley lines, but even a couple of examples will illustrate what I'm talking about.

The invention of forceps, for instance, was a very helpful thing for the few women who truly needed (and still need) help during birth. But their entrepreneurial inventors had quite an influence on birth history when they saw the potential to make profit and thus kept their design very secret so that midwives or families had to go to them directly for help. Sociologists and cultural anthropologists can tell you lots more about how the development of social status is partly linked with the holding of a certain kind of knowledge, skill or technology that others do not hold. They could also tell you about how, if you want to be even more successful, you need to go on to persuade more and more people that they need your knowledge, skill and/or technology. But the bottom line in relation to birth is that, if we respect nature, most women don't need technological help. (If we intervene or scare them, they may do, so let's not do that either).

Ultrasound is another good example of how technology has undermined women's knowledge. I'm not saying that this is 'bad' as a technology, because it can be incredibly useful, and I absolutely uphold every woman's right to use the technologies that are right for her. I just want to note that, as researchers like Sheila Kitzinger and Jo Murphy-Lawless have pointed out, before we had ultrasound, women were the main source of midwives' and doctors' knowledge of the pregnant baby. If we midwives wanted to know how a baby was doing, we had to ask the woman about the baby's movements or other aspects of its wellbeing.

Nowadays, the use of ultrasound (and other related technologies that let us 'look inside' the body) circumvents the need to ask women such things, and this can undermine a woman's sense that she holds useful knowledge about her baby. Which is a terrible shame, because there are things that women can know about their pregnancies and babies that no amount of any kind of technology can ever tell us – and let's not forget that, even though technology is amazingly clever and useful, it is also fallible and only as good as the person using it and the framework within which is it used. This doesn't mean we shouldn't use it, but I wish I could tell all women that their knowledge is just as valid, and sometimes more so.

2. Certain groups also profit from the idea that birth is risky and that their knowledge, technology, institution or protocol can reduce that risk.

Again, I'm not going to get all conspiracy theorist about it, and I don't want you to take my word for it because I think it is vital that we all think carefully about everything we hear and decide what resonates for us, but I think this one thing is worth bearing in mind when you encounter any ideas about birth.

There is, sadly, profit to be made from scaring women into thinking they are at risk and have to do certain things, or see certain people, or pay for certain services in order to keep themselves and their babies safe. This approach isn't just found in relation to birth; it's used almost everywhere. It's used to sell insurance and financial products, to persuade us to get our cars, boilers and bodies regularly checked and to get us to buy all sorts of things that we don't really need. The really interesting thing is that many of those who are on the 'selling' end of this idea truly also believe it themselves and genuinely think that what they are offering is the best and safest thing. I don't like the way in which fear is used to sell, whether it's done with intention or otherwise, and if you don't like it either, then you can decide – right now if you like – to refuse to be made to feel scared into making a particular decision, no matter how good the intentions of the 'seller'.

3. You know WAY more than you think you do.

Enough of the negative, because what I really, really want you to know is how amazing you are, and how amazing your body is, and how much you already know (even if you don't know it) and that you can trust yourself, your body and your baby. I have seen women crave weird foods that turned out to be exactly what their body and their baby needed for nourishment. I have seen women and babies work together to get the babies born in a way that best suited the situation. I have seen things that appear to be mysterious and/or miraculous, and each of them serves to build the awe in which I hold women's bodies and our ability to grow, birth and feed babies.

As a culture, we can sometimes be so arrogant about what we think we know through scientific and other modern ways of knowing. And these ways of knowing ARE amazing, and yet there are so many other amazing ways of knowing and kinds of knowledge – some ancient, some personal, some unique – that we will never learn by the means that are valued the most at this point in history. Yes, there are always situations where modern technology, knowledge and skills will be needed if everything is to turn out well, and we do need to respect nature and be aware of her wildness, but most of the time things will go well, women's bodies know what to do, babies know when and how to be born, and trust is a better guide than fear. Even the National Institute for Clinical Excellence began their recently revised intrapartum (labour and birth) guidance with the statement: *"Explain to both multiparous and nulliparous women who are at low risk of complications that giving birth is generally very safe for both the woman and her baby."* (NICE 2014).

In birth, as in life, there are no guarantees. It doesn't matter how many pinging machines we bring into the room, how many research studies we do or how many specially-trained people are standing around. They will never be able to prevent every problem. What they will do, however, is to continue to undermine women's knowledge, prevent the flow of the hormones that make birth happen (and generally happen pretty well) and perhaps cause problems that wouldn't have happened if we had left well alone.

My wish for all women and families is that we could move towards spending a bit less time applying monitors and risk assessment (which, as we now know from lots of research, don't help nearly as much as we thought they might) and put more of our time and energy into helping women understand, explore and honour their personal ways of knowing. Because birth is something that women and their loved ones have done for a really long time. It is about much more than the wriggling of a tiny body out of a larger one. When we birth, we don't just birth babies. We birth ourselves, we birth our families and we reshape our lives. Birth is a journey. I hope that this book has helped you to consider what is important to you on that journey and explore some tools and ideas which will help you find your way.

Also by Sara Wickham

Inducing Labour: making informed decisions

Sara's bestselling book explains the process of induction of labour and shares information from research studies, debates and women's, midwives' and doctors' experiences to help women and families get informed and decide what is right for them.

Group B Strep Explained

Explains everything that parents and birth workers need to know about Group B Strep; a common and usually harmless bacteria which can occasionally cause problems for babies. Sara discusses screening, preventative measures, alternatives and wider issues.

Vitamin K and the Newborn

Find out everything you need to know about vitamin K; why it's offered to newborn babies, why are there different viewpoints on it and what do parents need to know in order to make the decision that is right for them and their baby?

Birthing Your Placenta (with Nadine Edwards)

A popular book which helps parents, professionals and others to understand the process and the evidence relating to the birth of the placenta. No matter what kind of birth you are hoping for, this book will help you understand the issues and options.

101 tips for planning, writing and surviving your dissertation

These 101 tips are useful for students at any stage of their academic career. Written in an accessible, friendly style and seasoned with first-hand advice, this book combines sound, practical tips from an experienced academic with reminders of the value of creativity, chocolate and naps in your work.

PP to treat constipation:
- VITAMIN C POWDER
- MAGNESIUM SULFATE / CITRATE
→ a couple of days after birth